# HELPING
# OUR
# PARENTS

## How to be an Effective
## Healthcare Advocate

Michael J. Guy, J.D.

# CONTENTS

# Introduction

My wife, Jennie, and I were watching an episode of the television series *Blue Bloods* staring Tom Selleck. Selleck's character, Frank Regan, is the commissioner of the New York City Police Department. The Regans are portrayed as a very close, educated, successful and influential family. Even the grandson, a patrol officer, has a Harvard Law degree. Selleck's character and his father (played by Len Cariou) live in the same house. His father is a retired NYC police commissioner. They eat meals, watch sports, drink or talk about cop family matters in most of their scenes. In this episode, Selleck's TV dad has suffered a heart attack. Once gathered at the hospital, the doctor addresses the family, "first of all, I need a list of his medications." Police Commissioner Regan (Selleck) responds with, "I don't know. I should know this", which is delivered with a dimpled yet severe look of humbled frustration.

It was only a few seconds of a scene in a TV show, but it portrays where most of us are with the idea of helping our parents navigate the medical industry in their later years. When you have your *Magnum* medication list panic attack, anything you say or do other than immediately producing the requested current list is insufficient.[1]

Janet, my mother-in-law, spent over a year in the Boston Massa-chusetts medical centers while recovering from heart valve replace-ment surgery and its complications. During that time, Jennie pretty much moved to Boston and was with her mother every day.

Jennie really missed our dog, Deuce, and maybe me a little too. On the weekends, Deuce and I'd drive to Boston to see Jennie and Janet. As soon as I was within 20 feet of the nurses' station one or more of the staff would eagerly greet me and offer up where Jennie and Janet were in the facility and what they were doing.

While walking by that nurses' station and being instantly updated, I'd often see another person there to visit a loved one. "Is my mom still in room 304?" the family member would ask. "Let me check. What's her name?" was the typical response from the nurse typing at the keyboard. Which patient do you think receives the better care?

Because Jennie was there helping her mother, the folks in the hospital had a heightened awareness of Janet and thus were engaged with her care to a greater degree than other patients. I realize it's prob-ably not practical for you to put your entire life on hold and move to Boston, but there is much that you can do to fully engage the medical folks if you have the knowledge to correctly prepare and do the most with the time you have. Preparation and consistency are the keys to being an effective healthcare advocate.

You will work with medical professionals that will respect your efforts and, if you are truly effective, they will come to rely on you as a valuable part of your loved one's care. You will also find that you are going to be a major irritant to some in the medical industry and they will not be shy in letting you know it.

We can meticulously plan for our later years in fiscally responsible ways that have zero possibility of protecting us from the true frustrations of aging and illness. Our leaders create laws that are thousands of pages long, written in our nation's finest politically malleable legalese. Laws can't protect our parents' dignity in a medical facility or nursing home. The sad fact for the majority of us is that we will one day find ourselves tearfully exasperated and alone with one or more of our basic needs not being met for at least some period of time. It will not be the result of any form of intentional neglect or elder abuse. It will happen simply because when you are relying on others for care you are depending on human beings, overworked and imperfect, just like you. Don't let the insurance company, senior housing, skilled nursing or medical facility salesperson standing in front of the camera or in the glossy extra heavy stock literature fool you, they can't do a damn thing to insure that Dad will not someday be helpless, in need of care and stripped of his pride at some point. It does not matter how many times you tell yourself that his nursing home, hospital or rehabilitation facility is "the best". Regardless of their work ethic or workload, those caring for Dad know that ultimately a patient without someone to help them and monitor their care can wait longer.

Not everyone becomes permanently dependent on strangers. I am sure there are kind loving families that care for their loved ones in their family homes, bedside, with the warm and fuzzy feeling we had for the television Waltons. The vast majority of medical professionals and workers do sincerely care much more often than not and some even put forth a level of compassion that makes them the true living angels that they are. Sadly, families like the Waltons and angels are the exceptions. In Dad's moment of lonely realization, when his adult diaper is soaked, smelly and he just coughed up the cold tomato soup that he spilled the other half of on himself, the angel will be on vacation, on break, or having a bad day when he pushes that call button for the countless time in what is to him an eternity. Your loved one will never be the highest priority of anyone but you.

We don't plan for, or even think about, how it will be to see our parents, any loved one, or ourselves become increasingly vulnerable and dependent on others due to illness or simply the natural aging process. There may be nothing that we can do to truly prevent forms of human error, excusable neglect or even the outright abuse of every senior entrusted to the care of others. We do, however, have the power to stack the odds against it happening to our parents by getting involved in helping them manage their care, advocating for them, and caring for them with the loving compassion that we expect from others.

Productivity is crucial in any business, be it manufacturing, a non-profit food pantry or your local hospital. If a doctor and supporting staff can see more patients in a day, they are fiscally more productive. The result of that inevitable economic pressure is that when Mom goes to an appointment and the doctor comes in the room 30 minutes late, typing on a laptop, they are either completing notes on the patient they just left in the other room, hoping spell-check will help them to pronounce her name or locate the most recent test results in her file.

When you go to a meeting at work, you have to prepare and be ready to offer the best input you can. Doctors don't have that luxury in today's cost conscious medical environment. They have to quickly skim the most recent page and a half of Mom's records to refresh their memory, interpret test results, maybe do some form of examination, make critical treatment decisions, explain it all to her and hope to make something close to an accurate notation of the visit in the notes, all in roughly 20 minutes—while under the pressure of the several other folks sitting in rooms waiting to have him or her come into their room late typing on a laptop. What are the odds of your parents (or anyone) with two, three or more medical conditions, coming out of that appointment with a solid understanding of what's going on?

## What the Heck is Healthcare Advocacy?

Jennie and I were the primary caregivers for our parents from the time we became aware that they needed our help until they died. Three of them were able to die in their homes. In managing their medical care and the care of others, through short and long term illnesses, we have alternatively worked and jousted with medical workers, administrative individuals, insurance providers and family members. We have shared countless experiences, joyful and horrendous. Along the way we've accumulated a fair amount of practical experience for two laypeople functioning in the procedurally and technically complex medical industry.

Within a few months of opening our elder law office, we became aware of an unanticipated need that law school did not prepare me for. Clients would come in for an initial visit and we'd spend less than half of the time talking about elder law. Once the conversation turned to documents related to medical care, it grew to more than just "what paperwork do we need for Mom?" The clients we meet with have a thirst for knowledge that goes beyond having the correct estate planning documents in place and hoping to avoid selling the family home, camp and spending Mom and Dad's life savings to pay for long term care.

At some point while managing our folks' medical care, we started informally asking medical personnel, at all levels, for input on how to best help our loved ones. We talked with nurses, doctors, specialists, case managers, medical administrators, insurance professionals and the maintenance staff about how to help our parents. The response was enthusiastic and respectful from much of the medical community. All either said they have been such an advocate for their loved one(s) or they are prepared to be one when the time arrives. Healthcare advocacy by family members is needed and patients with effective family advocates receive better care. When asked how to best help Mom and Dad, nobody in the medical profession could tell us how to be a healthcare advocate, but they were clear that Mom and Dad need one.

We had taken copious notes of those conversations as well as amassing other healthcare related materials over the years. We went back to the boxes of paper and computer files, summarizing it all in an effort to create an outline or simple document to guide clients when helping their patents. It quickly turned into a bit of a research project. We assumed there had to be a wealth of material to guide folks on how to navigate the medical industry for Mom and Dad, information that we just did not know about.

We contacted area hospitals hoping to meet with them to discuss the process of helping our parents navigate the medical industry as they age and approach death, what we had started calling healthcare advocacy. Only one had the time. We were privileged to meet with several department heads and even the CEO of the organization. They provided excellent insight into the way they operated and their experiences with families trying to care for their elders. The information clearly helped us to define some of the paperwork issues that a budding advocate would have to deal with and we did hear their perspective on the family members' role in their parents' healthcare. Ultimately, we were able to validate the way we had cared for our folks and the material in our notes, but did not get a copy of that healthcare advocates' secret manual that we hoped for.

The next effort was to write many letters to geriatric and family medicine doctors. We received one response. It was from my parents' doctor who had retired at that point. She was very nice and gave me a good hour of her time.

I asked her about how family members should tactfully engage with doctors and nurses to help their parents understand and manage healthcare issues. It was clear the topic was foreign to her. After working to formulate an opinion, having been put on the spot, she settled on "Mike, you did a good job with your parents." She had seen that I went to appointments with them, explained things and was respectful of her staff. She had no idea that there was a plan in place and that I was not just giving Mom or Dad a ride to the office and sitting in during the visit.

She then volunteered a story about the end of her father's life, explaining that her father died from complications that could have been mitigated or avoided and that she wished she had engaged more in his care. I found it interesting that when trying to advise me as to the best way to help our elders navigate the medical industry that her mind would immediately go to a personal story that involved death, medical errors and her own regrets.

One of the letters went to my doctor. When I saw him several months later, he had the letter with him and we discussed it. He made comments on things like medical treatment paperwork and other things you'll read about later. He too volunteered a personal story. It was about the death of his mother that involved a challenge for him as the advocate.

His mother had been sick, it seemed like the end of her life was near and she could no longer make her own decisions. He knew his mother's choices for end of life care but the rest of the family was not so clear. There came a point when it was questionable as to whether a specific type of treatment would be something she would choose to have. The discussions escalated to the point that the only way the family could agree was to go on a treasure hunt for some document that could help them. Fortunately, they did find an old medical form in her house that was sufficient to settle the dispute.

Both medical professionals had on the tips of their tongues personal examples of the challenges that face someone who advocates for their parents' care but neither had a conscious awareness of what a healthcare advocate is. Everyone agrees with it, but nobody knows what it is or how to do it.

The next step in trying to find some clear direction on how to help folks effectively advocate for Mom and Dad was to start reading more than a few books, periodicals, journals and spending countless hours with online databases of all things medical and legal in an effort to learn what the professionals have to say on the subject. I did not find anything even close to a succinct guide for those of us trying to help our parents. There are many books about healthcare written in the self-help style to simplify and explain the medical system to laypeople like us. They are very accessible, written in easy to follow prose, packaged and marketed very attractively. They sell a lot of copies. Others are academic works of such density that you need a dictionary, a thesaurus, high-speed internet and a lot of coffee to get through the introduction. They don't sell a lot of copies. Don't be scared. The authors and readers of the academic material are safely tucked away in faraway places of higher learning.

The research provided some clues and the occasional tip for someone taking care of Mom and Dad, but not the advocates' handbook that we really need. The research then turned into a sort of healthcare advocacy reading of books, scholarly articles, and policy papers written by doctors, lawyers and nurses.

Most of the commentators seek to solve a big problem. Some call for a need to change the way doctors think, the way they are trained, or a global change in the way the business of healthcare operates. All of the issues are important but they have nothing to do with you not having Dad's medication list when the doctor asks for it. The issues they write about could someday, if corrected, help your parents but that's just too far removed from what they need now. Most of the problems these commentators bring up can be resolved (or worked around) at the Mom and Dad level, today, by an effective advocate. Healthcare advocacy will not fix the acknowledged problems with healthcare. It will help Mom and Dad, but it cannot be done by doctors, lawyers or medical workers with the next wave of trendy administrative titles on their business cards. You have to do it.

## Janet

The patient you'll be reading the most about is Janet, Jennie's mother. A retired teacher and breast cancer survivor, she was a most vibrant life force. More than anything, Janet loved her children and grandchildren. Having them around was about as good as it got in her world. When that was not possible, shopping and travel were good substitutes.

Janet suffered a long and complex series of illnesses. Life events aligned in such a way that Jennie was able to act as her primary healthcare advocate and caregiver in the years prior to her death. The complexities of Janet's conditions took them through multiple hospitals, over a year in an acute care rehabilitation hospital and close to a year of 24x7 hands-on care in Janet's home. Janet's story is the extreme. Most of us will never experience a fraction of what Janet endured, nor will we be a tenth of the advocate and caregiver that Jennie is. It is from the overwhelming enormity of their shared experiences that we have many good examples for you to read and learn from. There are several other characters in our stories, but Janet is the one you'll get to know the best.

## Jennie & Mike

We were born, raised, live and work in Kittery, Maine. Jennie is a retired civil service Human Resources/Administrative Officer. She is an experienced bookkeeper and legal secretary. I have worked in retail, as a bridge troll (gatekeeper on a drawbridge), founded and operated a small technology business and, for my mid-life crisis, went back to finish college and then to law school. Together, we operate an elder law office and teach classes in healthcare advocacy at local adult education programs.

While I may have compiled these words, every example of advocacy that shows model character, compassion and guts is all Jennie. The lessons learned would not be possible without her leadership.

The stories you'll read are true but most of names have been changed out of respect for the heroes' privacy and to protect the mediocre, the ignorant and the guilty.

The title was originally going to be *Helping Our Parents Die* but we thought it best to drop those last three letters. I didn't want to be mistaken as someone promoting their opinions regarding euthanasia or offering a punk perspective on end of life healthcare. The title was softened, but in a way, death is the end result of your work as Mom and Dad's advocate. If you take the time to truly get it right, you will improve their quality of life when they need you most, when they are old, sick and at the end of their lives. You really can help them die, or should I say, have a better death.

The purpose of the book is to provide a process for how to be an effective healthcare advocate for Mom and Dad. There are stories combined with light research that supports both our experiences and ideas. I have tried to make it accessible and somewhat entertaining. There is a lot to being effective at this. No matter how much or how little you can do, focus. Take the time to prepare and then be consistent in your efforts.

An unanticipated benefit of our efforts has been that we have enjoyed more meaningful relationships with the loved ones we've care for, a level of connection that we had no idea existed, one that we never would have experienced had we not taken the time to slow down and get involved with them, their care and their deaths.

We sincerely thank you for reading these words and hope they are useful as you help the ones you love. If you take the time to care for them with all the preparation, compassion, consistency and love you can muster, we assure you a tremendously meaningful and rewarding experience that will change you forever.

## Chapter One

...................................

# Why Advocate?

Dad slipped and fell coming up the steps on Thanksgiving Day. He was in his 70's and went straight down onto his tailbone. When Dad would fall he'd just want to sit there for awhile, to assess the damage. I ignorantly helped him up and it was clear, this was very painful.

We were prohibited from making the house, as the occupational therapy folks say, handicap-accessible. To Dad, if it appeared that a handicapped person lived there, it might in some way look poorly upon or even embarrass his family. He would not even allow a handicap plate on his car. After years of convincing, he did agree to the blue card with the wheelchair on it, hidden in the glove box, used only if it could make life easier for Mom.

Dad did not have a primary care provider (PCP) that he saw regularly nor had he ever gone to a local hospital. He carried very good family medical coverage through the retirement plan of his former employer. It was for Mom, and my brother and I when we were kids.

When he returned home from WWII, someone that Dad perceived as a person of authority told him that for his service, which included being shot down over Germany, months in a POW camp and the loss of his right leg, the government was going to take care of him for the rest of his life. That translated into a 220 mile round trip drive to the VA hospital in Togus, Maine whenever he needed a doctor.

In the days after the fall, Dad was in a lot of pain. He tried to take it easy, use alternating heat and cold on his back, and he took more VA pain killers than usual (they'd send him far more than he ever needed, so there was always a large inventory locked up in the basement). A week or so into December, he called for an appointment and drove to Togus. They X-rayed him, ultra sounded him and sent him home with instructions to take it easy, use heat and cold, and take more pain killers—as needed.

Through the holidays Dad was in pain but he put on a good front for the family. Come January, it's time to ride. Most local seniors head south. My folks went north for a month or so to ride around thousands of miles out in the woods on snowmobiles with others half their age. They loved it, a leftover pleasure from riding as a family when my brother and I were young. That season, Dad stayed at the lodge while the gang rode most of the time. It was assumed that he was aging and his back pain was just a part of the process.

Always a lanky man, he had lost 20 pounds and was looking gaunt, very unhealthy. Other than doing the taxes, explaining paperwork from time to time and mowing his lawn, Dad never seemed to require much from me as an adult. He dealt with the VA medical issues. If he did not understand something, he'd just roll with whatever they told him. After his Thanksgiving fall, it seemed important to hear what they had to say for myself. I wasn't sure what good I could do, but Dad reluctantly agreed to make another appointment and allow me to ride along.

The doctor reviewed the record and re x-rayed him. I asked about an MRI. They did not have one at that facility yet and we were told it was not needed. It was just the natural aging process and arthritis torturing his well worn body. It just did not make sense that it could be accelerated by a single event. Why would his pain level dramatically spike immediately after the fall if there was not something else going on? As it was curtly made clear to me several times, the tests were conclusive.

When we asked about having an MRI done outside of the VA we were smugly told that we could, if we wanted pay for it. They had no idea Dad had been paying for and ignoring access to local healthcare for more than 40 years.

When we asked about other VA facilities in New Hampshire and Massachusetts (much closer to home than Togus, Maine) that did have MRI machines, we were referred to the administrative folks who professionally condescended that we could but it would be a process. I was ready to carry through with the process, but Dad never wanted to rock the boat. He feared somehow that the man who promised his war-beaten, one-legged body care for life might get mad and change his mind. As for Dad's back, the firm VA position was "Degenerative condition, there's nothing more to be done. You need more meds?"

Eventually the pain was so great that he consented to go to the local hospital emergency room. He was given an MRI which uncovered

small cracks in the bones of his back. A few days later he had surgery
to correct the problems. By the following Thanksgiving, he had recov-
ered to the condition that he was before the fall and was able to cut
out the extra case of monthly pain pills. That winter he surprised the
sledding crew by going on most of the rides. He later confided that
between the extra medication and the pain, he could not remember
the previous year's riding season or much of the last year for that
matter.

Had I engaged with Dad's healthcare before things got critical, he
may not have had to lose a year of his life because of a medical facilities lack of technology and the staff's general mediocrity. I was not
knowledgeable of his conditions or their treatment and was ignorant
of what he needed. All I knew was that he had one leg, back pain and
went to the VA. I hadn't even tried.

### I'm Sorry, We've Done All That Can Be Done

Jennie's mom, Janet, had heart valve replacement surgery. Due to her
severe osteoporosis, her chest cavity bones essentially disintegrated
during surgery. There was no simple way to close the cavity when
the surgeon, Dr. McBride, was finished. The consensus was that they
would have one chance to close and they were not sure yet whether
they would have to operate on her heart again.

After two days, it was decided that no additional heart surgery
would be needed, but ten days later, her chest cavity remained open.
Her body was not producing enough of the type of blood cells (platelets) that stop bleeding and they could not close without a lot of
platelets. They were giving her blood transfusions and bags of pure

platelets to build her up for the procedure. The ICU team was watching and waiting for that short window of time when they could do the procedure to close.

Other than to go home for a shower and maybe a nap, Jennie had been at the hospital since the surgery. Early mornings she would go to the hospital chapel just outside the ICU doors to pray for her mother. Knowing that Dr. McBride would usually be coming by to see Janet before his day became hectic, she'd try to grab a few minutes of his time. It did not take long for him to start looking for her in the chapel. It was there, usually before 7AM, that he began to trust, rely on and work with Jennie as Janet's healthcare advocate. Jennie is not a medical professional, but he knew that she showed up, was clearly committed to her mother and was knowledgeable of Janet's medical history as no other. She also asked well thought out purposeful questions.

Throughout those post-surgery days, most of the medical staff reached the conclusion that all that could be done medically for Janet had been done. They get a look about them when they believe someone is dying. It's more somber (funereal?), but not unlike the look folks get when they just know the home team is losing, again. It's not that they give up, they've just seen these events unfold so many times that they can't help but resolve themselves to what they see as inevitable. Some of the medical staff won't easily make eye contact with you and others try too hard to console you with the understanding that your loved one is dying.

In his book, *The Secret Language of Doctors*, Dr. Brian Goldman writes about medical slang and the negative effect it can have on the culture of a provider organization. One of the slang terms he quotes is "failure to die". Dr. Goldman wrote that "failure to die implies that a patient's continued existence is utterly futile." Medical futility does not have a formal definition and "...doctors and nurses can only say that they know it when they see it", and that "all too often, medical futility is a judgment made by the health professional based on what he or she—not the patient—would want." [2] I do not know if there were any closed door, lunch room or smoke break conversations where the term failure to die was bantered about, but regardless of the slang used, the message projected to the family by our local hospital was clear, Janet's time had come.

Based on the position of the doctors and nurses, most of Janet's family and friends became very vocal that doing anything more to prolong her life was cruel and inhuman to Janet. The problem with that position was that it did not fit within Janet's choices for her end of life care. From the oldest documents in her file to the most recent, through all of her medical ordeals, Janet wanted all efforts made to keep her alive if there was any chance for her to be able to enjoy the company of her family a little longer.

Even Dr. McBride was starting to gaze at the floor when discussing Janet. In addition to her chest still being open and her body having to recover from this extremely invasive surgery, she had advanced loss of kidney function, osteoporosis, an undiagnosed blood issue preventing the generation of blood platelets, chronic obstructive pulmonary disease (COPD) and she was also on a respirator, without which, she could not breathe on her own. Closing her chest was one thing but she had a lot of other apparent impossibilities to overcome.

The opportunity came to close Janet's chest cavity. It was successful, but she quickly fell into a coma. It was a mystery to some and simply another unexplained circumstance in a lost battle to most.

There were several dialysis discussions. Janet's loss of kidney function had been on the edge of needing the treatments. They try to hold off on that because once you start, most are on it for the rest of their lives. Getting hooked up to a machine several times a week to have your blood cleaned you run the risk of infection and other issues, not to mention the dramatic change to your quality of life. After a day or so of debate between nephrology (dialysis folks) and the other groups, they started her on hemodialysis to help the kidneys do their job. A day later, she came out of the coma, but then they had to add three dialysis treatments a week to Janet's list of conditions, yet there was some joy in the shadows.

Janet was awake, eyes twinkling and able to enjoy the visits of her family. She knew what was going on, and soon was able to communicate with anyone who would take the time to understand her. It takes a lot of patience to have a conversation with a person who can't talk and is not in any condition to communicate other than with their eyes and a squeeze of your hand.

Janet had become a medically complex patient that did not fit into any of the check boxes on the insurance forms. The medical provider/insurance industry ecosystem has clear paths established that typically work well for both business models. Once the hospital can't show the insurance company a need for you to be where you are, you get discharged to increasingly less costly places and eventually, if all goes well, you get to go home. Janet's conditions dictated that she should be in ICU, the most expensive room in the hospital. It's not a place you stay very long and she had been there for several weeks.

Janet could not go into a regular hospital room. She was on a respirator, had multiple system failures, needed advanced monitoring and was getting three dialysis treatments a week. In discussions about Janet's eviction from ICU the administration blamed the insurance company, "this is an insurance rule", "this is not our decision", "I am sorry, it's just the way the system works." Fortunately, Jennie had the foresight to have Janet sign the required permissive waivers that allowed her to communicate with the hospital and insurance company on Janet's behalf well before the surgery.

It was clear that moving her anywhere in her current condition was a tremendous risk. The hospital agreed but insisted that it was required. What went unsaid was that the staff had decided that any additional time in ICU would be a waste of hospital resources.

Our initial conversations with the assigned insurance company case manager floored us. She had only some of the history of what had transpired since the surgery and a partial list of Janet's conditions. The insurance case manager was provided whatever the hospital case manger had time to assemble or felt was important. The insurance company did not believe us at first. It took several calls and asserting ourselves firmly between the hospital and insurance company case managers to make the entire situation clear.

This was not to be a remote circumstance. Throughout the remainder of Janet's life, discrepancies between the actual and the reported medical status would be a constant battle for us. The medical and insurance industries may have more technology than NASA, but they are either just too busy; simple interpersonal communication and accurate records transfers fail the cost effectiveness test; things just have a way of working out to support decisions on medical futility; or, it all comes down to some unspoken, path of least resistance method of getting where the administration needs to be.

The chain of information starts with the doctors and nurses who enter things into the system. Even if the latest technology is at your fingertips, when you're busy do you take the time to report all that you saw or thought of? A case manager assembles the records they deem important in compliance with procedure and sends them to the insurance company who in turn assigns it to one of their case managers who then tries to fit the case file data into the language of the insurance company's procedures and your insurance policy terms. Many decisions regarding our care are made by humans that do not regularly communicate with each other.

The insurance company has no reason to investigate what it receives unless there is some glaring weirdness or someone tells them they have incorrect information. They have no reason to believe the data sent to them is not an accurate representation of your loved one's situation.

The insurance company case manager, seeing the entire scope of Janet's condition, was able to keep her in the ICU for a little longer, but the locals were not very happy with our efforts.

We had reached the limits of our local hospital. It's a good facility, they have some rock stars, but Janet's care was dependent on more than that. The ICU folks still had that look. In their minds, it was just a matter of time, days, maybe hours, for Janet. We had gone to bat with the administrative folks and leveraged our insurance company to support Janet's choices, just as they had in their effort to make Janet's end of life decisions for her. They were fed up with us interfering with their business process flows and clashing with personal views. At some point, it occurred to us that we are only an hour from one of the world's great centers of medical knowledge, Boston, Massachusetts.

Janet could not walk or even be wheelchaired out to the car and driven to the emergency room of a major medical center. She would have to be transferred directly into a Boston ICU. If she went, it would be a major project, exponentially complicated by the need to coordinate the local hospital (with which the relationship was now strained to say the least), the insurance company and the extremely busy folks in Boston. There were heated discussions about Boston, both in the ICU and in several family meetings.

Nearly everyone was against Boston. The consensus was that everything possible had been done, that it was too dangerous and we should just make Janet comfortable and let the hand of fate take its course.

We had tried to cover all of the foreseeable scenarios with Janet before the surgery, but we had not talked about Boston. Jennie and I discussed her healthcare choices with her in detail many times and she was clear, she wanted everything to be done that was medically possible. Boston was the last hope to fulfill her wishes.

Most of us would have given up long before, willing to get the morphine and go to sleep. Not Janet. She wanted to fight and it was clear to us that her local hospital felt that they had done all that could be done. Janet was able to understand what was said to her, by us and the doctors. While she could not speak, she could communicate well enough to satisfy the doctors in charge. It was clear, she wanted to try Boston.

When Jennie first started advocating for Boston, our naivety was laughable. I am positive that many hospital employees did laugh at us. Suggesting that another facility might be able to achieve a different result was not only insane in their minds but also a major insult. The locals shut down on us in all but rudimentary communications.

Jennie tried working with the hospital case management team to get Janet placed in an appropriate Boston major medical center. She was constantly rebuffed by the medical staff and the administration, "there is nothing Boston can do that we can't." It did not take long to learn that major medical facilities just do not open their door to you simply because you want Mom sent there, especially the door to the ICU.

I'm sure many of the medical and administrative staff at the local hospital thought of it, but it was Jennie that advocated the blood issue. It was a documented fact that the locals could not do anything with Janet's low blood platelet issue in her condition and it only took a Google search to learn that Brigham and Women's Hospital (Brigham) in Boston might be able to. Combining the platelet mystery with her complex multi-system failures, the argument could be made that the resources of a major medical center/teaching hospital might be a medical necessity for Janet. The doctors and administration conceded the point, but dragged their heels. She was old and going to die soon anyway, what's the hurry?

Dr. McBride and Jennie had one of their early morning chapel meetings. Everyone was tired. Jennie tearfully pleaded, "have we gone too far? I don't know if I can do it. Should we keep fighting with everyone or just let Mom rest?" Shaking his head, "I'm sorry, I can't tell you what to do. I agree you're losing ground here." "What would you do, if she were your mother?" "I'd go to Brigham" was all he said while hugging her as he left the room.

That day Dr. McBride took time that he did not have to make

phone calls and meet with medical staff members and administrative heads. You could feel the tension in hallways and the ICU. By the end of the day tempers were flaring, but Janet was going to the ICU at Brigham.

Janet succeeded at Brigham and after 5 days in their ICU was transferred to an acute care rehabilitation hospital where, over many months, she was weaned from the respirator, learned to walk again and eventually returned home. Janet's choices were upheld due to Jennie's advocacy efforts for her mother. She was able to live another couple of years to enjoy her family, which is what she had asked for.

## Brigham

The reception in the Brigham & Woman's Hospital ICU is a bit of an overload. The ICU rooms are much smaller at Brigham. Janet arrived to a swarm of doctors and nurses. Not like you see on TV after some tragic event or violent crime, but more like hearing a super tight band cooking through an up tempo number that they're really comfortable with.

Every doctor, nurse and administrative person who came in knew all of Janet's conditions. All were sincerely and actively interested in Jennie's knowledge of her mother and gave her a business card. There was no search for who they should be talking to, everyone involved just knew. It was telepathic. At Brigham the employees were inquisitive and appreciative of Jennie where locally most were irritated by her, often disrespectful and always eager to find a less inconvenient family member to deal with. We were positive the local ICU had implemented "Code J" to warn doctors that she was on the floor. At

Brigham, they were giving out email addresses and phone extensions and, to our total amazement, they answered the phone or returned calls and emails promptly.

This was all happening in a place moving exponentially faster than the local hospital. If the locals did not have enough time in a shift to do all their work, how were these folks managing to do vastly more work in one and extract and utilize information from Jennie?

Janet had severe osteoporosis. The curve in her back looked like a question mark. That made it very painful for her to be in certain positions. Someone in Janet's condition has a lot of testing done. For you or me, being lifted and slid onto a hard surface for some imaging test might be uncomfortable. To Janet, it was excruciating. There are things that can be done to minimize her discomfort. Jennie often tried to forewarn the local staff of the issues with moving Janet. Those efforts were sternly met with, "you wait here", as Jennie watched Janet being wheeled out of the room with terror in her eyes. Remember, she could not tell you how much it hurt unless you made the effort to communicate with her, or noticed the tears. At Brigham, Jennie's concerns were addressed, heeded and appreciated.

Locally, Jennie was ushered out of the room at every opportunity. They allowed her to stay with Janet when she was given her medications and maybe when she was bathed, if she had been a good girl. Jennie was now allowed to be with Janet during nine out of ten examinations, procedures and tests.

At home, they'd tell Jennie to leave with a promise to come get her after. That rarely happened. Jennie usually had to keep jousting with the lady behind the security intercom to be allowed back at her mother's side. She learned a trick, ask someone else to speak into the machine. If they didn't hear Jennie's voice, they opened the door on the first try. Janet's desire to have Jennie there with her did not matter. In Boston, if Jennie was asked to leave, Janet was made to feel that everything was going to be ok and they came to get Jennie as soon as possible, without fail, as promised, for Janet.

You have seen TV hospital doctors doing "rounds." They go to see each patient and discuss what is going on regarding their care. Years ago, when your doctor used to (or was allowed by the insurance company) go to the hospital, they did it throughout the hospital, today it seems it's only done in the ICU. Locally, rounds are basically the morning change of shift. The doctor coming on duty walks around with the nurses that are coming on and going off shift. They stop in front of each door and recite the overnight vital signs of the patient from the night before, and any updates. Jennie would stand or sit near the door to hear what was being said. That was ok. Then she started asking questions and correcting facts. That was not ok. It wasn't long until they started closing the glass slider and cloth screen to keep Jennie out of the conversation or from reading their notes. At Brigham, once the staff became fully aware of Jennie's knowledge of Janet's medical history, they invited her to join in the rounds, every day.

Rounds at Brigham go a little differently. The group is larger, a lead doctor and a pack of interns fresh out of medical school. They don't run down the stats. Everyone involved is expected to know them. Jennie always did. The rounds consist of the lead asking questions of the residents and they not only had the answers but they were offering suggestions that he took seriously and sometimes he changed the care plan accordingly. This was a leading ICU specialist teaching and at the same time learning from sharp young minds that have just excelled at the finest medical educations in the world, all while leveraging Jennie's knowledge of Janet to improve her care. There was none of the condescension and derogatory energy that was experienced locally, it was the polar opposite.

One could read the previous few paragraphs as my merely bashing one hospital while kissing the collective ass of another. While there is some well deserved praise given, the reality is that, while the two hospitals used the same basic tool box, they could not have been more different.

If we make a list of just the mechanics of Janet's care from the two hospitals, they did not really do anything differently. They used the same tests and got the same results. The folks at Brigham did not resolve the platelet issue and in fact came to the same result as the locals. As the locals curtly condescended, Brigham did not uncover some undiagnosed issue or provide some medical magic beyond the scope of what they were doing.

Some could argue that Janet was on the verge of turning the corner for the better and she would have had the same result locally. I doubt it. They had written her off. In their minds she was heading from the ICU to the morgue. They had not even looked for a suitable rehabilitation facility that could accommodate her complex medical conditions. Sometimes it is not what you do, it's how you do it. That is the difference between local and Brigham.

The experience we had at our local hospital is the most difficult type imaginable for someone trying to help Mom when she is seriously ill. Jennie's efforts were constantly thwarted and countered. It is hard when the hospital culture wants you to shut the hell up and let the medically futile patient die. I do not know how Janet and Jennie did it.

Janet was alert and competent. She saw the way Jennie was treated day and night. Medical folks may have expensive degrees but they tend to forget that not being able to talk, or being old, does not always mean that you can't hear. She heard what was said about Jennie and her efforts. Janet had conditions that seemed insurmountable, she was under a lot of family stress and she was in a local hospital whose position was that she was a waste of their resources. It really was too much for anyone to handle. How could she possibly muster the superhuman effort to improve with the weight of her world literally coming down upon her? She was better off in the coma. Contrast that with an environment where the respect for Janet was put right up front by everyone who came into contact with her, respect that treated Jennie as a part of Janet's care. A place where she watches and listens to her daughter interact with the medical folks who actually value and utilize what is offered to improve her care. To Janet, it was an environment of healing as opposed to conflict. Her treatment choices were honored due to Jennie's advocacy efforts for her mother. At Brigham, Janet got a transplant. Her stress was replaced with hope and pride in herself. That is why she improved and is the difference between the two hospitals. Sadly, most moms do not experience a Brigham and still fewer have a Jennie.

It's easy to listen to the medical folks and submit to their personal views, as filtered through the science of medicine under the watchful eye of the administrative and insurance powers. It's very hard to make end of life decisions about Mom and not base them on our own choices and values. Advocating for a loved one's healthcare choices is not for wimps. Each of us has the right to have the healthcare choices we make upheld. We have an obligation to help our parents, to educate them about the medical questions, help them document their choices and make sure the family and the medical folks all know what they are.

Most of what goes wrong in medical facilities is caused by the same things that fail in any workplace. Perhaps it's an over simplification, but the things that make your job suck happen in hospitals too. It does not matter if we're talking sales, plumbing, engineering or healthcare, if those in charge allow an atmosphere of negativity towards the product, customer or patient, it will infect and ruin the culture of the organization and they are going to fail. We can't fix situations like the one at Janet's local hospital. We can learn to effectively advocate for Mom and Dad's choices and in doing so, improve the care they receive.

## Big Cheese in the Bus

Panic mode, struggling to keep up with the crew racing Janet from her room and into the ambulance, Jennie jumps in the back followed by Dr. Fitzgerald. To a very confused Jennie, Fitzgerald barks, "I'm going with you."

An attendant is doing what he does. Jennie is blue-bagging her mother. A blue bag is an emergency medical device that one uses to manually pump air into the lungs of a patient that can't breathe on their own. Fitzgerald is alternatively assertive to those he is directing and comforting to Janet and Jennie, as cool as they come. Cambridge traffic is beyond heavy. A Harvard graduation ceremony is letting out. Fitzgerald's slinging out directions, backseat-steering around snarls and jams. He's also on the phone updating his team at Massachusetts General Hospital (MGH). They're hustling together what's needed to get Janet breathing on her own again. She arrives, lights flashing, MGH does what they do and once again, it's not Janet's day to die.

Janet had been in an acute care rehabilitation hospital in Cambridge, MA. The reason she was in a rehab 70 miles from her home was their respiratory specialization. They were working to get her off the respirator and breathing on her own, or at least on an oxygen tank. They also have an in-house dialysis unit. Jennie has rented a room in nearby Somerville, MA. Most days, she's in the hospital when Janet awakens and leaves when exhausted or when Janet falls asleep for the night.

Janet, after completing a dialysis treatment, had been wheeled back to her room. While Janet ate her lunch, Jennie went out to get hers. Returning, as she stepped out of the elevator on Janet's floor, she heard the urgent alarms of code blue, code blue, room 372. Code blue means that something drastic has happened and the patient will die if they don't do something now. A patient can't breathe, their heart has stopped or both. Janet had aspirated. Aspiration occurs when someone takes food or liquid into their lungs. She could not breathe.

Jennie ran in the room as a nurse was yelling for help. Dr. Fitzgerald arrived third. Jennie grabbed the blue bag from the wall and started getting air into Janet. The next in was the ambulance EMT crew who happened to be on the floor after bringing someone in. Code blue means you go for a ride in an ambulance (if you're not already in a hospital). Two weeks prior, Janet had progressed to the point where she was off the respirator and was breathing on her own with the help of decreasing amounts of oxygen. The trachea opening in her throat where the respirator was connected had not healed up yet. The EMTs wanted to intubate her. That means put a tube down her throat to hook her to a respirator. Jennie screamed for them to stop. They argued policy. If a code blue is in effect, EMTs are in charge. The doctor on duty, Dr. Davey, was just watching it all unfold, not reacting or engaging. Jennie screamed louder, "MGH has experience with her multi-system failures and bleeding issues due to very low platelets, she needs to be transported there." Ignoring her, the EMTs moved toward intubation. Dr. Fitzgerald yelled the loudest, "Jennie's right, transport her as is stat!"

They both knew that, in spite of Janet's progress, having a person inexperienced with her complex conditions perform an emergency procedure was far more risky than a ride through the city with Jennie doing her breathing for her with the blue bag. With her blood clotting issues and the unknown status of the stoma (the existing opening in her throat), she could drown in her own blood on the way to MGH.

I can hear the medical folks out there crying foul that there is no way this could happen and absolutely no way in hell Jennie was allowed to ride in the ambulance and blue bag her mother. We'll, it did and she did.

Dr. Fitzgerald is the doctor in charge of the dialysis unit that cares for Janet, along with several other dialysis facilities in and around the city. There are many dialysis procedures done every day, and in many of them the buck stops with him. Some may see his face on occasion or even hear a kind word, but most patients never know who he is. As the months of rehab and dialysis passed, the communication between Dr. Fitzgerald, Jennie and Janet moved from occasional visual contact and maybe kind words to familiarity, conversation and eventually a first name basis.

Over time, Dr. Fitzgerald came to see that Jennie was more than the companion daughter. She was Janet's medical historian, a veritable answer sheet for any medical worker willing to listen, the one who speaks up when the pills are not the same ones as yesterday and the reason the call button gets answered. As with Dr. McBride back home, Dr. Fitzgerald was impressed. A level of mutual respect was attained and communication happened. It all culminated when the head of a prestigious kidney treatment group asserted himself and jumped into an ambulance to help a patient and her daughter. Janet was not his patient directly, but one of hundreds under the care of several levels of dialysis nurses and doctors under his supervision. He could not possibly offer the level of attention that he bestowed on Janet that day to every patient. The odds of Dr. Fitzgerald being on her floor at that time when they needed him are almost lottery-like. However, on that day Janet's real good fortune was Dr. Fitzgerald and Jennie. Without Jennie's advocacy efforts, the connection between Dr. Fitzgerald and Janet would not have been what it was. He would not have been as aware of Janet's history and conditions had Jennie not facilitated putting her mother closer to the forefront of his mind than the majority of his patients. Without her past efforts, he would never have been comfortable allowing Jennie to jump in during Janet's time of crisis.

## It's Not Just Us

In his book, *How Doctor's Think*, Dr. Jerome Groopman dedicates an entire chapter to the story of a character named Rachel Stein and her daughter, Shira Stein. Rachel, a successful business professional and former seminary student, adopted Shira from an orphanage in Vietnam. Shira had serious health issues from the time she came to the United States. The infant spent a month under the care of leading doctors in Boston Children's Hospital, most of it in the pediatric ICU. She could not eat or drink and whatever was wrong with her was causing her body to not process oxygen properly. Every advanced technology was used to help her breathe, but nothing seemed to consistently help. The team of doctors eliminated one diagnosis after another. All they seemed to know for sure was that something was causing a serious form of pneumonia. The diagnosis that was settled on was Severe Combined Immunodeficiency Disorder (SCID). Indicators of SCID include a low T-cell count. T-cells are important to our body's ability to fight off disease. The treatment that was prescribed was a bone marrow transplant. Dr. Groopman described it as the "most extreme measure in medicine to cure a disease." Shira then mysteriously improved enough to be transferred from the ICU to a regular hospital room, but the diagnosis remained and the bone marrow transplant was on the schedule.

Rachel researched the disease well. As a layperson, it appeared to her that Shira's symptoms did not check all the boxes perfectly for SCID. She asked intelligent questions of the doctors and they acknowledged that Shira had an atypical case of SCID. Rachel developed and advocated for her own diagnosis, an undiagnosed nutritional deficiency that was causing the low T-cell count. The doctors had the blinders on, were trenched in on the SCID diagnosis and moving rapidly toward the bone marrow transplant. Rachel was rational and assertive, but not getting anywhere. The medical staff felt that Rachel's effort was that of just another justifiably pained parent (and layperson). To them, her diagnosis was without clinical merit. Rachel wanted the T-cells and other things tested again before the transplant and they did not want to do it. In their minds they had conclusive evidence that Shira had SCID. She argued that Shira, as an atypical case, was a research opportunity for the hospital and that an additional set of data could only support whatever major breakthrough that might follow. It worked. They agreed to the additional testing. It showed a normal T-cell count and pretty much a normal kid. She was home with her mother in a few days.[3]

Dr. Groopman utilized a full 30 pages in his book about the limitations of how doctors are trained to think and how that leads to the mistakes they make for the story of Rachel Stein. At the same time, he has provided a great example of effective healthcare advocacy.

One of the books that Dr. Ira Byock has written, is entitled, *The Best Care Possible*. In it he tells the story of a daughter caring for her mother. Michelle is portrayed as a very diligent Manhattan professional that is quite capable of advocating for her mother who suffers Alzheimer's and lives in a nursing home in Florida.

Michelle wanted to do all that she could to effectively advocate for her mom from her home in New York City, it was recommended that she meet with the doctor at the nursing home to set up "contingency plans" that would establish controls over her mother's care. As a result of her efforts, her mom's medical documents (healthcare advance directive) clearly indicated that the care plan was to provide comfort and quality of life for her mother rather than put her through senseless medical procedures without Michelle's consent.

In the face of the documents on file, her mother was transported to a hospital following a bout of vomiting where a battery of tests were done, she was bruised from IVs, more confused and scared than usual and a hospitalist (hospital staff doctor) was talking about treatments for a possible diagnosis of cancer. The healthcare advance directive was clear. That should not have happened. The nursing home directions were for Michelle to be called before anything outside of the care plan was to be done. A newly hired nursing home doctor had not taken the time to read the file or the care plan. None of the staff experienced with her mother bothered to speak up.[4]

In both Dr. Groopman and Dr. Byock's stories, we have two intelligent, successful and professional women going through extremely frustrating and emotionally draining experiences. Rachel's story had a relatively happy ending and Michelle's ended in frustration. Both women did all that they could based on what they knew about the medical industry and healthcare advocacy.

Rachel was there present with her daughter in the hospital. Michelle was 1200 miles away from her mother. It is not the distance that thwarted Michelle's efforts. As you will read, regardless of where you sit, you have to be engaged in the process of advocating. Putting documents in place is only the first step. Preparation is part of it, but without a consistent pattern of engaging with the providers, your planning will fail.

People just park their parents in nursing homes all the time. They visit once in a while. Like a crock pot, set and forget. I don't believe

Michelle did that. She did the best she knew how to do. She made sure the documents were correctly in place to protect her mother's best interest. The problem for her mom was that almost all of the other residents of the nursing home had been parked there to simmer alone and, overall, the staff behaves accordingly. Michelle, through regular communications with the rest of staff, should have known about the new doctor and established a dialog with him. Doing so may not have guaranteed a different result but it certainly would have drastically reduced the odds of it happening.

The common thread in the stories you have read and will read in this book is that without help from someone, your medical care will not be as good as it could be. Not everyone who gets involved in their loved ones' healthcare saves a life, solves a puzzle that the best doctors do not on a given day, or eliminates great pain. Sometimes, we just make it easier for Mom and Dad by going to appointments with them, providing information and being a second set of ears.

## Not the Practice of Medicine

Once you have prepared and start to get involved as your parents' healthcare advocate, you'll have medical workers asking you if you are a nurse, doctor or what exactly it is that you do. The more effective you are, the more you'll hear it. Some in the industry, maybe even your friends and family, will be snippy and claim that you have no business helping your parents with medical things because you are not a doctor or nurse. Ignore them. You don't need a medical degree to help Mom and Dad.

There is a local nurse who has created somewhat of a media

presence. We contacted her a couple years ago thinking she might be a voice for what we had labeled healthcare advocacy. Her response was that family members could not be advocates for their loved ones because there was no oversight or state licensing involved. She'd didn't get it. There is no state licensing board for parents who advocate for their children's healthcare and this is no different. Actually, it's the logical continuation of our parents caring for us when we were young.

When discussing our care at the end of our lives Dr. Ira Byock wrote that "Only the need to control symptoms is uniquely medical. The more basic needs are broader than the scope of medicine."[5] Dr. Byock is telling us that your effort at being Mom and Dad's advocate is not the practice of medicine and as such, you are as qualified as anyone else to help them. The truth is that, with all that you know about them, you're very likely the most qualified. As a healthcare advocate, you'll learn a few medical words, but you won't be practicing medicine. The medical folks can't do what you can.

## Chapter Two

........................

# Be the Medical Historian

### *Never saw it coming*

J anet should have had knee replacement surgery on both knees 10 years prior, but she had places to go, people to see and shopping to do. Contrary to her extremely youthful spirit, putting it off was slowing her down to the point where painful mobility was quickly becoming pain without mobility. Janet and her children had been talking about knees for years. They had interviewed doctors while trying to work around holidays and travel to find the best time to do it. The years had passed and now it had to be done. Jennie lived the closest and had the most flexible schedule. She offered to help take her to the pre-knee surgery appointments and act as a second set of ears.

Jennie and her siblings each helped Janet with medical issues from time to time, but overall Janet managed her own healthcare. There was no reason for her not to. As Janet would say, she "still had her bean." A competent, educated and intelligent woman, she could make her own decisions.

From past encounters, Jennie had good reason to be concerned with Dr. Marie's role as primary care provider. She exuded a seamless aura of condescension buffered by intermittent half-smiles, far too busy to answer pointless questions from laypeople. Janet and the other family members didn't share Jennie's concern. Changing doctors was not an option. Because of Dr. Marie, Jennie engaged with Janet's medical care beyond merely going with her to appointments. She collected copies of Janet's medical records, all of them. She then studied them, looking up what she did not understand as she went. She then made copious outlines, notes and summary sheets. Jennie also had the foresight to contact the insurance companies, submitting the correct documents required for her to work with them on Janet's behalf and had the paperwork prepared to allow her to communicate with Janet's doctor's and their administrative employees. We had no idea how invaluable it would be in the years to come.

While deciphering twenty plus years of medical notes, Jennie noticed that twelve years back there was a mention of a heart murmur and an EKG heart test. Janet had no knowledge of any heart issue and had no memory of having been treated for it. The records did not show a prognosis, follow-up tests or any a further mention of it. A breast cancer survivor with kidney issues, chronic pain in both her knees and severe osteoporosis, Janet went to doctors often and had all sorts of tests done far more frequently than most of us, but nowhere was there any other mention of a heart issue.

Janet had been complaining of being tired. She could not bring in all the groceries from her car without sitting down for a few minutes and would often fall asleep with the rest of the bags still in the car. She reported shortness of breath and trouble getting winded on only a few stairs. Her claims were dismissed as natural aging and possibly a side effect of the medication she was taking for the chronic pain in her knees and back.

Jennie called Dr. Marie and asked her about the heart murmur and was told that it was not an issue, it would not affect her knee surgery and not to worry about it. Lacking confidence, she made an appointment for Janet with a cardiologist.

The resulting appointments and testing revealed major blockage in a valve of her heart. It was also learned for the first time that she was suffering from chronic obstructive pulmonary disease (COPD). The prognosis was that if she did not have valve replacement surgery, there was less than a 20% chance that she would be alive in a year. She was then referred to a heart surgeon, Dr. McBride.

The Friday morning of the surgery, her kidney function was too low and the operation was rescheduled for Monday. They kept her over the weekend and hooked her up to a heart monitor. It revealed that Janet's condition was even worse than previous testing had shown. There were dramatic instabilities in the opening and closing of her heart valve.

Despite all the pre-surgery tests and doctors' opinions, Dr. Mc-Bride told Janet's family after the operation that once the surgery started, they found the condition of the heart far worse than was expected based on all previous testing, including the poor results from the heart monitoring over the weekend. If they had not done the operation, she would have died in a matter of weeks.

It's not hard to find the lesson here. Maybe the pre-surgery testing for the knees would have uncovered the oversight, but we do not know that it would have in time. Jennie's acquiring and learning what was in all of Janet's records was a key to her success as the healthcare advocate from day one. We were amazed that something like a history of a heart irregularity could just fall through the cracks, but we had no way of foreseeing how that initial research into those records would time and time again provide the knowledge Jennie needed to be effective.

## What do you mean he's dying?

Late Sunday afternoon, the pain in Dad's back had become unbearable. We brought him to the local hospital and he was admitted. Scheduled for the next morning was the MRI that would reveal the damage to his back. The night before, all the doctors knew was that he was a male in his mid seventies, that he had physically declined over the last six months, had lost noticeable weight, appeared gaunt, claimed to be in much pain and that we, the family, thought it had something to do with his back. Suspecting that any coordination of efforts between the VA and a local hospital would either be impossible or take years, I naively provided the intake nurse a six-inch stack of VA medical reports that they were not going to even scan into the system, let alone read. I did not even have a list of his medications with me.

The blood work and initial tests came back around 10pm. By the time the doctor on duty had digested the test results it was close to midnight. With a somber face he had me sit down and told me that

Dad was dying and might not be going home. He explained what hospice was and suggested I talk to the rest of the family about it. In addition to Dad's pain, the tests showed problems in his blood and kidneys. I cried and Dad consoled me saying that it was going to happen sooner or later. He calmingly stated that he had enjoyed a good life and was ok with dying, all with a big smile and a look of near relief.

It didn't make sense. Dad hurt his back. The VA could not help him. We brought him somewhere else and now he is going under hospice care dying of kidney failure? A doctor had said it, one with many years of experience. He had forgotten more about medicine than I would ever know. He had the medical degree, a hospital full of technology and other doctors to support his decisions. All I knew was what I had seen my dad go through in the last few months. It did not feel right, but what other choice did I have other than to accept it?

The next morning I met with our family. They got mad at me, cried, got mad at me again, calmed down and then started to accept the fact that Dad was dying.

By the time we got to the hospital, the MRI was complete and a new Monday morning shift of nurses and doctors were buzzing around. A different doctor met with us in a small room. Guess what? Dad's not dying. My family thought I was nuts and got mad at me yet again.

Dad's back had cracks in some of the bones that they could fix surgically. He was anemic and that could be addressed with medications. His kidneys, while not 100%, were not that bad for a man in his 70s. He did die of kidney failure, 10 years later.

If I had compiled, knew the contents of and carried with me

a short summary of just Dad's recent VA medical records and an updated medications list, as Jennie did for Janet, I could have provided useful information to the Sunday night doctor and my dad may not have had to spend a night alone in a strange place having just learned that he is dying and I would not have put the rest of the family through the needless drama.

## Helen

The story of Jennie's finding Janet's lost heart condition is the extreme example. Helen was my mother's best friend for 75 years. When Mom died, I inherited Helen. Helen had hydrocephalus (excess fluid around her brain) and Parkinson's disease. In advocating for Helen there were many times where simply knowing her conditions and medication history saved her discomfort and the medical people taking care of her time and money. Hydrocephalus is not something busy medical folks deal with everyday. In Helen's case, the treatment of it meant that there were some imaging tests that she could not have done. The hydrocephalus was all over her records, but the new medical person (nurse, CNA, doctor, radiation technician or neurologist) in the office never has time to read the record. They like to do imaging tests on Parkinson's patients. Many times I found myself not just telling them that she had hydrocephalus but also asking them to double check to make sure she could have an MRI. I was never once condescended to or vented at for telling them something that may have prevented a medical error. Even if someone was a bit miffed at my interjection, it would quickly turn into appreciation of my input.

Parkinson's patients have their medications changed as the disease progresses. Neurologists come and go. The new ones don't have time to review the old medications. Several times, by knowing not just the current medication list but the ones that had been prescribed in the past, I was able to provide information that helped the doctor.

If you tell a medical worker that one medicine was tried and did not work or caused a reaction of some sort, don't expect them to thank you. You're only another source of information for them, they just keep on moving. Don't be disappointed, you will not get any credit but you saved your loved one some time, money and maybe some discomfort. You will also have saved the medical provider time and the insurance company money, which nobody will ever notice.

⌒

Dr. Angelo E. Volandes, in *The Conversation*, wrote that "The health care system is teeming with brilliant scientists, but there is a dearth of effective communicators and advocates." In his 10 years of undergraduate and graduate education, he received about one day of training on how to talk with patients. That means he had little or no training in how to communicate with patients before he started treating them. He also wrote that "Medical schools place far more importance on the capacity of applicants to show expertise in scientific reasoning, mathematical skills and memorization at the expense of the ability to communicate."[6]

Dr. Jay Katz was also a law professor. He was a great proponent of a patient's rights and the doctor's duty to provide the information that we all need to make informed decisions about our healthcare. In *The Silent World of Doctor and Patient,* he wrote that "Physicians are well trained to attend caringly to patients physical needs. Their education has not prepared them to attend caringly to patient's decision making needs."[7]

Most of the young people coming out of medical school have very few life experiences outside of academia. Where do young doctors get a chance to hone the interpersonal skills needed to communicate with your mom (who is old enough to be his or her grandmother) about complex medical and emotional end of life issues?

The communication breakdown between medical folks and patients is not limited to laypersons. In his book, *Being Mortal*, Dr. Atul Gawande tells the story of his father's interaction with a neurosurgeon. Dr. Gawande is a surgeon, his father was also a doctor. He had been recently diagnosed with a rare and difficult to treat spinal cord tumor. Dr. Gawande's father had some detailed questions for his potential surgeon who "was fine with the first couple (questions). But after that he grew exasperated. He had the air of the renowned professor he was—authoritative, self-certain, and busy with things to do."[8] Dr. Gawande's description of that doctor on that day is far more tactful, respectful and diplomatic than mine would have been. His story depicts two doctors that together could not communicate with one of their peers. If that surgeon did not have the time for questions from folks that speak fluent medical jargon, how much patience will he or she have for them coming from your mother?

In his Forward to the 2002 republication of Dr. Katz's, *The Silent World of Doctor and Patient*, the respected law professor Alexander Morgan Capron wrote that "…it is for the coming generation of physicians—along with lawyers, philosophers and social scientists to… break down barriers to mutual trust and true communication in the physician-patient relationship."[9] I'm sure that Professor Capron, Dr. Katz and the other commentators are correct. Improved communication is needed and if affected, will indeed improve healthcare, but Mom needs your help now. Until the medical folks agree to and implement a global change of the medical industry, you're just going to have to step up and facilitate meaningful communication between Mom and the medical workers treating her.

As Mom and Dad's advocate you are going to be constantly challenged by ineffective communication and sometimes you're going to be faced with medical workers that are not even willing to try. The medical folks know medicine, Mom and you don't. They have clinical experience and scientific knowledge that they are trying to apply and you know everything else about your mother. They have a job to do and it will seem as if it never involves what you have learned about her over the last 4 or 5 decades. One of you has to find a way of turning those two knowledge bases into some form of communication that benefits Mom and it's not likely to be the one wearing scrubs.

You're never going to know a fraction of what they know about medicine and you have no experience. You can't even pronounce the words they use and just when you learn some, they'll start using different ones. What can you possibly do? You can help them by providing information important to Dad's care that they don't have when they need it. You need to be the medical historian.

## Step One—Get the Medical Records, All of Them

Make a list of all of your loved one's current and past medical providers and get their records from them. It is not unusual for a doctor or specialist to work with more than one organization or even multiple groups within an organization and they may all have different medical records filing systems. They also move from practice to practice, companies and groups get bought, merge and then go out of business. Try to get them all.

You will be amazed at what you'll read when you start digging in. You'll see dates that conflict, records of other patients in Mom's file, procedures that are not done on women and more copies of discharge papers from the same visit or procedure than you knew could fit in one file.

Do not even think about fixing the stupid stuff. Everyone knows that your mom did not have a vasectomy, don't waste your time and energy, or anyone else's, correcting the foolishness. The records are not Mom and Dad's credit report.

The processes of getting medical records will vary as will the number of hoops they'll make you jump through. It all depends upon the individual provider's procedures combined with the level of competency and overall work ethic of the folks working in the medical records department. There's a lot of federal and state law on medical records. I hope you won't have to learn any of it. The bottom line is that everyone has a right to all their records under federal law and providers can charge you for them. The states set the amounts that can be charged.

Asking for electronic records on a CD will almost always be less costly than paper hard copies. Just to be clear, the records are stored electronically but you still need to ask for them specifically on a CD. If you don't request the CD, some companies will print them because they can charge you more for the paper.

Providers do not have to charge for the records and many that we have dealt with don't. It's not just the smaller providers, we've seen records from major medical centers come to us quickly and without any charge. If some or all of Mom's providers outsource medical records management to some out-of-state mega-data repository, you may wait longer to get them and end up paying more.

In preparation for Janet's return home from her short time at Brigham and lengthy stay in the Cambridge rehabilitation hospital, Jennie thought it might be a good idea to get all of the medical records from the heart valve replacement surgery onward to make sure she had everything before heading home to deal with the doctors there. The rehab and Brigham provided them within a week. Jennie wrote a letter to the mega-data repository that keeps records for the medical conglomerate that owns the local hospital that performed the surgery to request her file. Jennie knew to ask for the records on CD. About a month later an envelope with some CDs arrived with a bill for $1,260.00. When we called them on the fact that we had requested electronic copies and that we thought they were only allowed to charge us for a reasonable amount of time to make the CDs.[10] They responded by dropping the charge to $0, they didn't even bill for postage. Was that a one-time mistake by someone working for the mega-repository contracted by the conglomerate owner of the local hospital or a computer generated attempt at collecting free money from the innocent, unsuspecting and uninformed? We'll never know. Be a good scout, be prepared.

Each provider will have an authorization/release form or two and if they outsource medical records, that company's customer service bots may have some for you too. To actually get the forms, call each provider, tell them who you are and that you're helping Mom or Dad get copies of their medical records and ask for the required forms. Once you have the forms, fill them out and make sure you keep copies of everything. You may well end up having to request records more than once.

You want these records requests to come from your parents. Have Mom and Dad each sign their forms. Draft a cover letter and have them sign that also. Make sure the cover letter explains that they are not changing doctors and that they simply want to see what their records say. We've seen providers just assume you are asking for records because you're changing doctors and then cancel appointments and prescription refills.

You have a much better chance of getting the records quickly and free if the providers think Mom and Dad are asking for their own records. If you have to get them from the providers yourself, ask them what you need for documentation to do so. Use the same type of cover letter as you would if Mom or Dad could sign themselves. You never, ever, under any circumstances want a third party (especially not a lawyer) to request them for this purpose. All kinds of alarms go off, months pass, the number of pages you actually receive goes down and the price goes up.

Providers are not required to keep records forever. Every state that I know of has a medical records retention law. You may find that Dad's providers send whatever they have. If the retention law is 10 years in your state, you may get records going back 25 or more years but all they have to provide is whatever the law requires. Don't worry if you only get 10 years or so. You're mostly concerned with what has transpired in the years leading up to the point where Mom and Dad need you as their advocate.

## Step Two–Organize

If providers send paper records, copy them. Put the paper copies sent to you back in the envelope they came in and work from copies. Print out copies of those records that came on CDs (don't bother printing X-ray and electronic imaging pictures, but make sure you print the doctor's reports about them). You want one clean copy to set aside and one to markup and organize.

Put all the copies on the table and organize them in reverse chronological order (newest on top). Go through them and pull out all the duplicate records. Cull out any that are not the records of your loved one. Yes, you will find strangers in there.

Once you have removed the superfluous records and have them in reverse chronological order, it's time to start analyzing. We want to work toward having a usable summary that you know inside and out. You'll need to identify:

- **Dates**
- **Test results**
- **Reports on test results**
- **Medications (Past/Current)**
- **Admission records**
- **Discharge summaries**

I find it easiest to just go through them all slowly once or twice with highlighters looking for the important points before starting to type my notes and outline. If you use a different color highlighter for visit notes, test results, current medications, past medications and admissions/discharges it makes the sorting easier. Coloring is fun.

There are going to be some big words that you do not know, maybe more than a few. Don't be intimidated. Just take it one word at a time and Google them. You don't have to make the unfamiliar terms part of your daily vocabulary. You just have to know what they mean for as long as it takes you to craft your own meaning of them within the context of Mom and Dad for your notes. Hydrocephalus was hard for me to remember when dealing with Helen's medical folks, so I just said water on the brain. It was never a problem. Actually, when I did remember hydrocephalus, I'd get blank looks more times than not.

Depending on how thorough you are and how many pages of history you have to work with, your notes may well be quite long. That's ok. If you end up with several (or more) pages, you will also need to make a short one or two page outline of your notes. Do not lose track of the long versions though. This process of highlighting the records, writing your notes and then outlining them creates a format that will be easy for you to use when dealing with medical folks. Do not take shortcuts, the more pages of history you have the more time it's going to take for you to become familiar with the important facts. Throughout the process of organizing the records, highlighting, note taking and outlining, you are learning the medical history as well as summarizing it.

## Step Three–The Medication List

You will need a document with all of Mom's current medications, with the exact name and spelling of the medicines as it is on the bottles, the dosages, who prescribed them and when. You will need a second list of all of the medications she has taken in the past. That information should be in your notes and outlines from the medical records. Don't forget to include the date Mom started taking each one, the dosages, who prescribed them, any reactions with other drugs or side effects and when she stopped taking them and why.

## Step Four—The Brown Bag Test

Doctor's used to call it the *brown bag test,* maybe they still do. It's not just the list of prescription medications, it's a comprehensive list of everything in Mom and Dad's house that they take or might take. They used to ask folks to put them all in a brown paper bag and bring them in. The idea was to find all the prescription and over the counter things they take or could take, including antacids, vitamins, supplements, cough and cold stuff and anything else you can think of. You're in a position to be far more accurate than the brown bag test. You can go to their house and look through all the places that they will forget to look but will remember when they want one of those pain pills from when they hurt something back in the 70's or those ear drops that worked so well on you when you were 6.

Doctors can sometimes learn as much from what your father takes each day as they can by relying on him to relay symptoms. There can easily be interactions between prescription and over the counter items.

Don't be surprised at what you'll find in the back of drawers, cabinets, and under sinks. If the Father John's, feminine products, over-the-counter and prescription drugs, eye-of-newt and contraceptives from the last century are out of date, get rid of them.

All of the brown bag items need to go on the bottom of the medication list, especially the in date eye-of-newt.

## Step Five–Keep Up

Once you have your notes and outlines completed, you're done with the most labor intensive part of becoming an effective advocate. You've just created your most useful tool. You don't want to have to do that again. As you go to appointments with Dad, get copies of that visit's notes and keep them in reverse chronological order along with the other medical records. Don't forget to update your notes and outline with changes to his conditions, care and medications as you go.

## Step Six–Take Your Own Notes

When you go to your Mom and Dad's appointments with them, do not let the medical folks keep you out of the conversation. You may have to leave during some parts of your mom's examination, but you need to be there with her for all discussions with the doctor or their staff. Take your own notes and compare them to the doctor's notes afterward. You'll occasionally be surprised at the differences between what you heard from the doctors mouth, wrote in your notes and what you read on the official notes of the visit.

## Step Seven–Use Your Devices

Today's world of smart phones, tablets and carbon fiber zero-gravity laptops devices can be a huge help. You can carry paper around in a fancy leather folio if you like, but, do yourself a favor and put your research library in your devices and up on your cloud as well.

## How to be the Medical Historian

You're going to take whatever you digest from this book and fit it into your situation, lifestyle and personality. You'll appropriate the things you like and either ignore or spin the rest of it to fit your needs. I understand that, but one of the few things that I do know to be true of everyone's advocacy efforts and it is that diplomacy works and weapons of mass destruction do not. You will achieve greater success with a respectful and tactful demeanor when dealing with the medical folks. That is not to say that you should not assert yourself when need be, but yelling, demanding and generally being an ass will only hurt Mom's care and assure your failure as her advocate. You need to be Gandhi as opposed to your favorite evil autocratic historical figure.

Your knowledge as the medical historian is useless until someone wants or needs it. Even with your detailed summary and outline of the medical records, you're still a peon in the medical world. You're a little kid wanting to help Dad work on the car. You need to stand and watch for a while and wait for an opportunity to help. If Dad drops a wrench, pick it up for him. If the doctor suggests a treatment that has been tried before or a medication that Dad is allergic too, tell them. If you're not asked or don't hear something contrary to your knowledge of your father and his medical history, do not interject your ignorance. If your instinct tells you something is wrong, don't blurt out an uninformed statement. Ask a question. When you get to the chapters on how to advocate you'll read more about the kinds of questions as well as when and why to ask them (Chapter 7).

Never, ever call yourself the medical historian (or the healthcare advocate). They are your super powers. They don't need to be stated and they'll speak for themselves when needed. You'll know when it's time to utilize what you know about Mom and her medical history. It's like the frustration of paying every year for AAA, it all makes perfect sense when your daughter needs it.

⁓

Other than her last few years, my mom, Priscilla, led a remarkably healthy life. Her medical history contained little detail and no surprises. Jennie's mom was clearly a different story. She had a slew of conditions going back decades and had been on more different types of medications than most pharmacies keep in stock.

The more complex the loved one's medical history, the greater the initial workload will be. Don't rush it. Take your time and get the medical history summary perfect. As you will see, in addition to being your most useful tool, the preparation of the medical records summary is your healthcare advocacy training camp.

## Chapter Three

................................

# More than Paper

In the ICU and at most nurses' stations there is a white board (or flat screen monitor). It has the patients name, room number and treatment specific information. Some of the detail you might read on this board will be regular updates of vital signs, notes on nutrition and various things particular to your loved one. In bold print there will be a clear indication of what the patient wants done if they stop breathing, their heart stops or both. When that happens, and they try to save you, it's called resuscitation. If you don't want them to try to restart your heart or help you breathe, a doctor has to sign a do not resuscitate order (DNR). If you don't have a DNR, or other signed doctor's orders, you are 'full code', meaning that they will do everything medically necessary to resuscitate you until someone with the proper authority tells them to stop. That includes the use of cardio pulmonary resuscitation (CPR), including breathing devices like the blue bag or a respirator and those automated external defibrillator (AED) paddles that they zap people with to restart the heart (as seen on TV).

## She'll Never Notice

It had been close to two years since Jennie had taken Janet to Boston. After her days in the Brigham and Woman's ICU, she spent several months in an acute care rehabilitation hospital and then returned to her house in Maine with well managed home care. Janet had suffered a setback and was once again back in the dreaded local ICU.

Jennie left the hospital early on the 3rd of July and returned late the next afternoon. She needed a break and being a holiday weekend, friends and other family would be visiting Janet in abundance. I made an effort at a nice dinner. The next day we slept in with Deuce, our dog, took a walk on the beach and went for a motorcycle ride (Deuce doesn't ride). It was less than 24 hours, but it felt like a vacation.

When Jennie got back to the hospital, Janet was still groggy on the anesthesia from a procedure done a couple days ago. With her kidney issues, it would always take longer for her body to process medications. She was awake enough to smile and show us the twinkle in her eyes. After hugs and updates on the lobsters we had for dinner, the beach and Deuce ( Janet was not a fan of motorcycles either) it was clear that she was nodding off to sleep, the fog had not yet cleared. I headed home and Jennie went to the ICU desk to get updated on what transpired overnight. There it was, in bold red letters next to Janet's name, "DNR". Jennie immediately went to find the ICU doctor on duty. She found Dr. O'Toole, "my mother is not a DNR". He snapped back, "I know that". "Then why does it say DNR on the board!" He, to prove her wrong and her hoping to be wrong, they marched to the desk. A quick check of the last 24 hours revealed that a temporary holiday weekend fill-in doctor, Dr. Khane, had signed the DNR and placed it in Janet's file. It was signed by a doctor. It could not easily be changed without Janet's consent and another doctor's signature.

Still slowly coming out of her anesthesia induced stupor, she did not have the capacity to make such a decision, or to reverse it. In spite of all Jennie's efforts of the last few years to fulfill Janet's wishes, for the first time, if she had a medical emergency that involved her heart stopping or she was unable to breathe, nothing would be done to save her. That was directly against everything she had ever signed and every conversation we or her providers had with her about what she wanted with regard to end of life decisions.

Over time, we had acquired some useful phone numbers. I called the medical director's cell. If he calls you back in a few days, it might be a worthy topic. The callback came in less than 5 minutes.

While I was working on getting a meeting together with those involved, Jennie hunted down Dr. Khane. She quizzed him and he said that Janet had a visit from friends, family members and clergy late the previous evening. He stated that, "the family and Janet do not want her heart to be electrically shocked and restarted." Jennie asked if he tried to call her or anyone else about the change or if he had read any of her other documents on file. He did not and he had not. Jennie then asked how Janet could be totally unconscious from anesthesia 36 hours ago and clearly out of it that morning and yet somehow have the clarity to agree to a DNR against her wishes of the past 30 months. He responded "I am the doctor, she now has a DNR" and left the room.

The ensuing family meeting could easily have been a Jerry Springer highlight film. The facts of how Janet came to be a DNR were never discussed. The others were very vocal that Janet had "been through enough", doing anything more to keep her alive was inhuman and it was time to let her "die a natural death." The phrase "die with dignity" was paraded around. The medical staff was not on our side. They stoked the fire, explaining in detail how painful CPR is, that ribs are broken and the AED (paddles) are extremely painful. Then it became all about what some were calling "electric shock treatments" and that Janet should not have any. The lay people in the room did not understand the words being used and the medical professionals were fine massaging the family into negating Janet's choices and Jennie's efforts to adhere to them.

All logic and decorum had left the building. I tried to ask if the patient feels pain when they're unconscious during an AED zap and recited some quotes I had researched on the subject and was verbally blown out of the room. The line was clear and the one person whose voice mattered was still unconscious to the point of not being able to offer any input.

The only argument that made a dent in their effort was continually asking, "what does Janet want?" To which we always got a response of what others wanted or thought Janet should want. While Janet had been a physically very sick woman, other than when sedated, she was still sharp as a tack. Many heated debates about Janet's care were settled by simply asking Janet, as it should be. The meeting ended with the understanding that when Janet became alert enough, the medical director would interview her to decide if she was medically competent and whether she wanted DNR status or not.

After the meeting, due to the adversarial nature of the day, we waited for the rest of the family and friends to visit Janet and clear out before we went in. Janet was the Energizer bunny, her timing impeccable. By the time we got in to see her that afternoon the fog had cleared and she was 90% back. Able to understand and communicate with us, she was shocked at what had happened and we could not get the medical director in fast enough for her. He brought another administrator with him, a member of the clergy with a law degree. Jennie and I were not allowed in the room. Janet's DNR was replaced with a full code order. That was to be the last time that she was allowed to express and have her end of life choices honored.

Janet's Advance Directive named Jennie as her agent and medical contact. Everyone in the hospital knew Janet's choices for end of life care. Jennie should have been called before anything as drastic as changing Janet's status to DNR happened. They had called Jennie countless times in the past for far less.

The medical staff had decided that Janet was once again a medically futile patient and any further efforts beyond making her comfortable would be a waste of resources. Those caring for her used the illusion of authority to impose their views on her family. A staff member was able to influence one of Janet's children to say that they wanted Janet to have a DNR, Dr. Khane signed it and everyone else looked on, nodding in approval. They knew Janet's choices for end of life care, decided they were more qualified to make those decisions and facilitated changing them when Janet and Jennie were sleeping. The result of that wrongful exercise of authority was that Janet's rights were violated and she was given DNR status against her will.

If Janet did not have an effective advocate in Jennie, the DNR would have been placed in Janet's file, nobody would have told her it had been put there and when she had an event that required resuscitation, the medical personnel caring for Janet would have done their best to make her comfortable while she died. The scary part about that scenario is that everyone involved would have been fine with it.

Most of us would not choose to fight as long, nor as hard and against such increasingly impossible odds. Regardless, Janet's choices were inexcusably ignored when the end of her life was rewritten by others.

## The More Advocates the Better, Right?

Nobody had the flexibility in their lives that Jennie did. Others had young children and responsibilities precluding them from taking close to three years out of their lives to advocate for Janet. Jennie worked for two lawyers as a bookkeeper and legal secretary but, of the family, she was the one able to move things around to make it work. Because Jennie would be the one on site the majority of the time, it made sense to put her name on the documents as the agent, proxy, and in any other terms, the contact person for the providers, insurance company and the person making decisions for Janet when she couldn't. It was not any indication of preference of one child over another. It was simply the logistical choice. Jennie was not getting any privilege, just the stress. Documents were executed under the laws of Maine and Massachusetts, not New Hampshire (where Janet was a patient in the local hospital ICU) but there had never been a question of Jennie's role.

From the time that Jennie discovered the lost heart issue in Janet's medical records until well after her death, no one else had any interest in working with the insurance company, resolving all of the billing issues, being trained to manage her medical issues (enabling her to go home vs. a nursing home), acting as a caregiver for Janet, finding and managing those needed for her home care, helping her pay her bills or even doing her grocery shopping. Everyone was fine with Jennie's role as Janet's advocate, caregiver and personal assistant until she clashed with the medical industry.

When in Boston, Jennie and Janet were more than an hour away from most of Janet's friends and family members. An hour is just enough distance for everyone to be comfortable with Jennie advocating for Janet. Now however, the local hospital staff, family and friends were fed up with Jennie being, as they saw it, "in charge and bossing everyone around." They were working to get her removed from office. Remember, Janet was still making her own decisions, but they were often fired from Jennie's mouth and that was a huge irritant. It all came to a head when a minor decision had to be made as to Janet's care, all the family members were not consulted (it was not required), Jennie vocalized Janet's choice and all hell broke loose. The alliance of family, friends and medical workers mounted an attack on Jennie's authority to advocate for Janet. Janet was devastated, scared, and Jennie was discouraged to the point of breaking.

Healthcare advance directives ask you to name an agent, they may use different terms but the job is the same, to make decisions for you when you can't, and sometimes when you can. Maine's document provides a mechanism for your advocate (agent) to speak for you at all times, not just when you lack the capacity to speak for yourself. Janet was laying in an ICU bed in New Hampshire. Their laws about advance directives do not give agents the same flexibility. Under New Hampshire law, the agent is not allowed to make decisions for the patient until a doctor has ruled them to lack the capacity to make their own decisions. We have to remember that when Jennie spoke for Janet, she was not making the actual decisions on her care—she was merely reciting Janet's choices and stating what was already documented in her advance directive.

It was that difference between the two state's laws that the local administration leveraged in their first attempt to remove Jennie from her role as advocate. The result of the hospital's manipulative interpretation of state law was that if they ruled Janet to have the medical capacity to make her own decisions, the staff was empowered to ignore Jennie.

Jennie was not always seen by the local staff, family members and friends as an effective advocate. To most, she was an irritant, the cause of extra work and an interruption in the way things are done. They had never seen someone fight for a patient's rights like that. It was not normal. Something must be wrong with Jennie. The popular reasoning was that Jennie was a control freak and that Janet did not really want Jennie as her advocate and was somehow wrongfully influenced by Jennie. In other words, it was the conclusion of some that when Jennie expressed Janet's wishes they were not her true wishes. When Janet told them they were wrong, they chose to not believe her.

To test the theory, in the face of Janet's cognitive expression of her wishes and several years of consistent documentation requesting that Jennie be present during any medical procedures and decisions, nurses and doctors began making decisions with Janet behind closed doors, excluding Jennie, because they ruled Janet to have the capacity to make decisions herself. What Janet wanted, once again, did not matter.

Janet was scared and very nervous at suddenly going from having

Jennie at her side explaining things to being questioned by medical folks who very efficiently sought the answer they wanted or had time to hear. Doctors and nurses can explain things in terms we understand or be as technically obtuse as they have the time or are in the mood for. Sometimes she was a little ashamed to admit she did not understand what was being said or was simply too intimidated to speak up. The staff was most comfortable that Janet had the capacity to make her own decisions, understood them and there was no need for the irritating daughter.

Now Jennie had to hear what was going to happen, or worse, what had happened second hand. It all usually ended in a showdown in Janet's room with Jennie, the medical workers and often family and friends at which Janet would be informed by Jennie and questioned by everyone else. This happened with everything from the simplest medication change on up. Nothing changed in her care other than Janet being forced to watch everyone constantly fighting. Do not forget, Jennie was not making decisions for Janet, she was helping Janet to understand the questions. It was exhausting for Jennie, a massive waste of staff time and worst of all, torturous to Janet. In a few days, the drama subsided and the medical workers loosened Jennie's collar. Allowing her in the room when decisions were being made was more efficient than all the fuss of dealing with her after the fact. All Janet wanted was to get home to her house and have her family around her.

In their next attempt at negating Jennie, Janet was the pawn. She was asked, in the presence of her immediate family, if she wanted one or all of her children to be listed as agents for her on her advance directive. Janet knew the consequences. Regardless of the fact that her very right to manage her own healthcare was at stake, she could not, with everyone staring at her, find it in her heart to pick what she feared others might possibly see as favoring one child over the others. She desperately wanted her children to stop fighting and play nice together and her last attempt at making that happen was to sign a new New Hampshire Healthcare Power of Attorney naming all of them as agents. The hospital facilitated the signing of the new document on the spot, immediately. They had it filled out in advance with witnesses ready, pens in hand (with spares) at the door. Being an odd number of agents, if Janet was deemed to not have the capacity to make her own decisions, Jennie was out voted. Whether or not Janet had the capacity to decide was up to the doctors.

Most healthcare documents of this sort name one agent. If you have more than one, they'll never agree on the color of the blanket to be put on the loved one's bed. New Hampshire law allows for more than one agent, but they fix the potential conflict by stating that the first name on the document makes the decision when the agents can't agree unless there are other specific instructions (the law says nothing about voting).[11] Jennie had signed first. Technically, Jennie had priority and was still able to advocate for Janet's wishes as she had been. The local hospital administration, medical staff and the family did not like that part of the law, so they ignored it.

From the moment the new Advance Directive was signed, Janet's capacity was never addressed, she had it, but all decisions were put to a vote without her input. It was as if the new advance directive immediately empowered everyone involved to ignore Janet's choices for end of life care. The New Hampshire advance directive form provides questions about life support and has places to document end of life choices. At the signing, we asked about those sections on the form and were told "they're not important now" and those questions were left blank. Now the hospital could work with others that could be influenced to the make the decisions that those caring for Janet thought were best. With the patient's documented choices for care and the pain-in-the-butt daughter out of the way, they could get back to business.

## How Is That Even Possible?

I bet you're wondering what was wrong with the local hospital, maybe thinking that what you've just read is not believable or you're curious about how all of that could have happened. Part of it is simply that 'business as usual' in the medical industry is not prepared for healthcare advocates. The greater issue is that the medical documents (advance directives) that our lawyers and doctors give us to sign are insufficient when it comes to helping us define our true choices regarding healthcare when we're sick and at the end of our lives. There is also no assurance that the choices we make will be adhered to. Those are complicated problems and I doubt the medical and legal folks are ever to going to correct them. The good news is that if you advocate effectively, help them make informed decisions about their care and document them properly, stories like the ones you're reading are far less likely to happen to your parents.

I firmly believe that on a daily basis medical workers use their knowledge as power to manipulate patients and families to make the medical decisions they have deemed best in accordance with their clinical experience and training, combined with, administrative and insurance provider policies all filtered through their personal views

and prejudices. I don't believe it is done maliciously. It's the path of
least resistance to getting the job done and I doubt if it's always done
consciously. If I am correct, why don't we hear more about this issue?
I know they're two over used clichés and I use too many of them, but:
You can't see the forest for the trees; and, No harm, no foul.

I was fortunate to have the perspective I did while these stories
were occurring and was somehow persistent enough to spend more
than two years analyzing and researching how this medical power
play comes to be and is allowed to exist. Janet was my mother-in-law.
That is different than being my mother. I am not sure that had she
been my mother that I would have been able to step back and look
at what transpired as an observer.

Being a middle aged man with over three decades of conducting
business under my expanding waistline, I've gotten pretty good at
reading people. I was privileged to be able to watch Jennie interact
with the medical folks and participate in, while observing, the interactions between Jennie, the medical staff and the rest of the family.
With my collection of observations, I then worked to sort them out
and find material to test my conclusions. To be honest, I was shocked
to find the large amount of information that I did and I'm sure that
I haven't even scratched the surface of how the imbalance of knowledge affects the decisions we make as patients. Like Waldo, once you
start looking, he's everywhere.

Our stories of Janet's care are dramatic and far from the norm.
They were seriously exacerbated by the fact that Janet had Jennie, an
effective and engaged advocate. Without Jennie, this all would have
played out under the cover of darkness, unspoken yet effective patient management. Most of the time the influence exerted over your

care is truly harmless. You need the damn flu shot. Telling you that there could be side effects or that it may not work is not really that important in the scheme of things. Medical workers are like us. When we get busy, we cut corners. The challenge is to recognize when efficiency becomes a violation of patient rights.

In the *Introduction*, you read that the medical professionals acknowledge a need for healthcare advocates but can't tell us how to be one. That is because discussing how they advocated (or will advocate) for their mother and father and telling us how to do it for our parents are two different questions in their minds. One is a personal effort they see a need for and are proud to take on for their loved ones. They will lovingly put forth a greater effort at doing what they are trained to do because their connection to the patient is different, it's family. Helping their Mom and Dad involves additional emotions, challenges and a level of commitment that is not required for other patients. Asking them how to advocate for someone else's loved one causes a short circuit in the back of their heads somewhere. They are confident that their parents need an advocate, but they have reason to pause at the idea of every patient having one. Business as usual is not good enough for their Mom and Dad, but instinctively, they feel that it is for everyone else.

Think about what you do for a living. Regardless of whatever your job is, you do it differently for Mom. If the practice at work is anything less than what you believe to be perfect, things get done at a higher level when you're doing it for Mom or Dad. Even if "we do it the same for everyone", the level of attention goes up and you don't care how long it takes to do it for Dad. The medical folks don't put forth less of an effort at work when they're caring for your Mom they just do more for theirs, like you would.

⌒

The medical staff, family, friends and Jennie all had disparate opinions on what should and shouldn't be done to best serve Janet. Every person sincerely believed that they wanted what was best for Janet. The problem was that "best for Janet" was defined by each of their personal values, life experiences and knowledge (or lack of).

Janet's family and friends, including Jennie, felt that Janet had been through so much and they all wanted her suffering to end. It was overwhelming. Nobody involved can be faulted for feeling the way they did or the positions they took.

The medical staff and the administration were not doing anything different than they would with any other patient. They had concluded that doing anything other than making Janet comfortable and letting her die was medically futile, a waste of their time and of hospital resources.

Family and friends wanted efforts to prolong Janet's life stopped quite simply because they were exhausted, tired of watching Janet suffer and, as most are when dealing with the end of a parent's life, easily influenced by the personal values, opinions and priorities of the hospital workers, as employees and individuals.

In *The Silent World of Doctor and Patient*, Dr. Jay Katz discusses the doctor's role in patient care decision making. He observed that "Sociologists of medicine have singled out two criteria as central to the definition of a profession: the possession of esoteric and abstract knowledge and freedom from lay control." The sociologists are telling us that those trained in a profession think that you do not need to know what they do and that Mom should not have the ultimate say in her care. Those treating Mom and Dad were trained in, or at least frequently exposed to, the idea that you can't possibly understand the scientific and clinical aspects of medicine and that you need to stay out of decisions about your parents care. The majority of medical professionals that we've encountered do not indicate that to be their conscious belief. It does however help to explain why some medical professionals may act as they do and, combined with the economic pressures that hospitals are under and the family members' emotional or traumatized state of the moment, does shed some light on how Janet's wishes for end of life care were so easily allowed to be changed from what she expressed to what others felt she should have expressed.

Dr. Katz goes on to tell us that "doctors generally agree that patients do not have the capacity to participate in the decision making process." When doctors act on behalf of patients "identities become obliterated and only the doctor's voice emerges." The patient's wishes for care (and, if you're not careful, your efforts at advocating for them) combine with the doctor's opinion and, "collapse into one identity and one single authoritative voice emerges—the physicians. It alone pierces the silence and gives orders, without a need to explain the art and science of medicine or the physician's personal and professional convictions." If you have not seen this play out, you will. What Dr. Katz so eloquently described was illustrated when Dr. Khane ended his DNR discussion with Jennie by stating "I am the doctor, she now has a DNR" and walking away. You will see it when a doctor comes in to see your Dad and immediately starts pontificating in medical techno-babble in such a way that both of you are intimidated to the point of not asking questions or have no clue what to ask. Everybody is shell-shocked. That leaves only one voice in the room, the good doctor becomes the commanding authority, which gets him or her where they want to go efficiently and provides for a little ego masturbation along the way. Cost effective, enjoyable and professionally justified.[12]

In *She'll Never Notice*, the staff of the local hospital leveraged family to impose their choices for the end of Janet's life on her and in *The More Advocates the Better, Right?*, they pressured Janet to agree to a new advance directive as a way to permanently solve what they saw as a problem. They labeled the problem "Jennie", but she was not it. The dramatic events in those two stories are rooted in the fact that the nature of medical professionalism clashes with the purpose of healthcare advocacy.

Jennie and I worked very hard to support Janet's choices for end of life care, but how did she come to make them? Yes, they were defined by Janet's word and signature on many documents of legal priority, but that does not fully explore how an educated competent person came to make decisions that resulted in her undergoing every conceivable treatment at such a cost to herself.

The vast majority of people make their end of life care decisions from a position of ignorance, or at least seriously lacking the knowledge needed to make informed decisions. We are easily influenced by the media, the medical and insurance industries, religious figures, family members and we are too lazy to go beyond whatever cursory information our doctors (and lawyers) are capable of or are willing to take the time to provide. That is not to say that making decisions based on any of those sources are the wrong ones, they're just not fully informed, personalized or derived from anything close to independent thinking and as such, a disservice to ourselves. After reading about Janet's choices, most folks would not make the same ones. They would not choose to pursue life to that extent. Doing so, as a knee jerk reaction to the stories like the ones in this book, is a mistake that many have made. There are far more individuals out there that have made severe decisions in fear of a quality of existence that they have not fully defined. People sign documents that place limits on their care that, had they been informed, they may never have otherwise consented too.

For most of us, the healthcare decisions document (healthcare advance directive) is either something thrown in by your lawyer when you sign your will or (if you bought the deluxe package) the trust(s) that are a part of your estate plan. If not, it was, or will be, slid in front of you to sign when you're really sick, old or both by a medical worker. Most of us sign when we're scared or really stressed from signing another stack of papers that we don't really understand.

Doctors give me the impression that, along with a person's Will, Powers of Attorney and other legal documents, they think the lawyers are providing the healthcare advance directive and related forms. I can see where they get that idea. Lawyers have been including basic versions of them with the estate planning packages they sell for decades. The lawyers assume that the doctors are doing the rest of it because, well, they're doctors. The result is that nobody is taking ownership of helping us to make informed choices.

When I started critically reading the medical documents that medical groups and states produce, I was curious why they choose the questions they did. The medical and legal folks have simplified it for us to the extent that they think necessary, but I have to wonder if the efforts to make it simple were not based, at least subconsciously, in the reality of their professions. If they don't think we can understand the medical language or that they should not have to bother to explain it to us, did that in some way result in an oversimplification of the forms? Does the reality of medicine as an industry influence the questions? Regardless, the forms (and their instructions) that I have read fail to empower folks to make informed decisions about healthcare and end of life choices.

If the advance directive given to you to sign has any questions or check-box options regarding the specifics of your care, they will be, directly or indirectly, about limiting your care when the medical folks have decided that any further treatment would be futile. It may address issues of dementia, pain management, life support and other things, but every question will lack specificity and because of that, can be interpreted to support decisions of medical futility.

When the vast majority of us hear the term life support, our minds immediately flash to the human vegetable, the unfortunate soul who lies there zombie-like with absolutely no hope to ever regain consciousness. That image is clear in our minds when we're filling in the check boxes on the advance directive form at the hospital, in the doctor's office or when we're signing our wills with our lawyers. When you are asked to sign an advance directive, they will not discuss the circumstances surrounding you potentially being on life support or even what they mean by life support. It will all be done with the understanding that if medical events align in such a way that you end up existing as a human vegetable, that you want the plug pulled. *Pulling the plug* is not a medical term. It is an image in your mind. The medical folks have the ability to correct any mis-understandings that you and your family have, or they can passively allow you your delusions.

Go back to that vision of the human vegetable, the one we dread, the reason we're signing the form without really understanding what it says. What if you're on life support and not a vegetable? You are alert and able to communicate with others. Perhaps you're only tem-porarily unable to make your own decisions, as when Janet was still waking up from the anesthesia and they slid the DNR into her file. If that scenario plays out for you, how do you know that your family won't just follow ideals and opinions of the medical folks?

The forms do not get specific, explain in detail the implications of the medical issues, any other choices available to you, why you might want them or provide anywhere near enough information for you to make truly informed choices. The result is that you have signed a vague document that can be interpreted as those reading it see fit. Your providers have it documented that, if you're on life support, you want the plug pulled. The definition of life support and every other aspect of your care will be decided based on how it gets explained to, or is inflicted on, your family by the staff at your local hospital.

Justifications for the simplicity of these documents are that we don't care or are incapable of understanding anything more detailed. That may be true for some, but I'd wager that more than a few of us would engage in making more informed choices on the specifics of our care when we're sick or at the end of our lives if anybody both-ered to tell us there was more to be done.

In 2015, the American Journal of Public Health published an article entitled, *The Myth Regarding the High Cost of End-of-Life Care.*

It discussed the fact that some sources say that as much as 13% of the cost of all medical care nationally is spent on those in the last year of their lives. The article opens with "Healthcare reform debate is largely focused on the highly concentrated healthcare costs among a small portion of the population and policy proposals to identify and target this high-cost group." They are saying that the idea that we're spending too much money on folks during the last year of their lives is a large part of the ongoing efforts to fix our healthcare system. That translates into powerful efforts to not spend money when the medical workers decide there is nothing left to be done for folks that they deem to be medically futile and in the last year of their lives. In closing, it is written that "Maximizing Value (i.e., increasing quality while reducing costs) in the care of high-cost, seriously ill individuals is a major public health challenge facing the nation's health care system and economy." When you read a statement like "increasing quality while reducing costs" in a policy document, you know that by the time those words get to the hospital floor, where your Dad is, all that the pay grade actually treating him is dealing with are meetings, memos and supervisors aimed at getting that DNR up on the whiteboard.[13]

In *The Secret Language of Doctors*, Dr. Goldman wrote in the context of the medical workers ability to communicate about end of life care and decisions that "Talking is not enough; the challenge is to get patients and family members to understand the options well enough to make an informed choice."[14] Dr. Goldman was writing about actual end of life choices when someone is dying. I would argue that, if done in the best way possible, this needs to done by way of educated planning and documentation well in advance of that, "there's nothing more we can do" conversation at the hospital.

We are not going to change the way the medical folks do their jobs. They are going to effectively inflict their opinions and business models on patients and families that have not taken the time to truly understand our end of life care options. If we don't bother or care, letting well educated policy makers, through the training, experience and personal views of those caring for us, make our decisions for us is probably for the best. However, if you are going to be an effective advocate for your parents, you need to have the ability to inform Mom and Dad about the importance of how the choices they make now will affect them later.

There are really only two positions to take when planning for our care at the end of our lives. We can hold onto every precious minute of our lives, as Janet did when she choose to never give up fighting death in the hopes of a miracle so that she could be with her family longer. Janet's position was pure, and clearly defined. Her wish to be with her family, as long as possible, was more important to her than any pain and suffering. Those that choose differently do not want medical science to extend their lives to the point that they end up existing rather than living. They do not want to be here if they're not going to have a quality of life that is acceptable to them. The problem is that we are given no instruction on how to define the quality of life we are willing to accept or document it in such a way that it gives our family and everyone caring for us clear direction.

The process of documenting Mom and Dad's wishes for medical care when they are old, sick and at the end of their lives clearly involves more than filling out forms. It is taking the time to learn what the questions are, what the possible answers are and being able to have meaningful conversations with your loved ones.

How do you bring it up? Where do you start? There are dents on every surface of the Buick and Dad's not even thinking about giving up driving. How the heck are you going to talk to him about his wishes for care at the end of his life?

Keep in mind that this is a process and everything you do while preparing to be Mom's advocate, from becoming the medical historian to making sure the correct paperwork is in place is part of helping Mom to define her true wishes regarding healthcare leading up to and at the end of her life.

Following the steps in the next chapter will enable you to help Mom put in place a healthcare advance directive that represents her informed choices regarding her medical care and gives the family, as well as those treating her, clearer direction regarding those choices. As you'll see, it happens through a series of little conversations as opposed to one very big one that nobody wants to have. The more uncomfortable you and Mom are talking about dying, the more you're going to like how this all works.

## Chapter Four

..................................

# Informed Healthcare Choices

M y mother and father believed that intravenous (IV) hydration is a major form of life support, on the same level as a respirator, the iron lung and a feeding tube. Some healthcare advance directives ask if you want artificial hydration (an IV in your arm) in the context of life support. An IV is also used for many other things. Most folk's mental image of life support is a person existing as a vegetable. Because nobody explains it to us and we don't ask questions, we make ignorant assumptions, check the boxes on the form and end up with Mom thinking that all IVs protract the existence of sleeping zombies.

You only have to go to the hospital once after Mom or Dad has a fall to know that many seniors are constantly dehydrated and always get an IV while waiting those long hours through the shift-change so that they can get X-rayed, imaged or whatever they do to diagnose a broken hip. Priscilla, my mom, only had one such hospital visit. She was a very cheerful advanced Alzheimer's patient and was just happy for all the attention. She got an IV. I knew she did not want an IV for the wrong reasons and did not tell the hospital of her true wishes. It was all in her advance directive (she actually wrote in the document "no IV ever"), which was on file at the hospital. Nobody looked. Talking to me was easier. Why was it ok for me to ignore my mother's wishes regarding treatment but unfathomable for Jennie and I to do anything other than fight tooth and nail for Janet's?

When I failed to tell the folks at the hospital that Mom did not want an IV, it was no different than a doctor providing only the information needed to get a family to make decisions about Dad's care that they think are best. I was just as ignorant and as big a violator of my mother's rights as Dr. Khane was of Janet's when he conspired with the medical staff, hospital administration and family member(s) to slide a DNR into Janet's folder when nobody was looking.

One could argue that I was only protecting Mom and it was the right thing to do. The problem with that logic is that when a doctor sells you a DNR, or your family colludes with the hospital staff to get one up on the white board while you're asleep, they too are doing what they think is best. It is a violation of her right to control her own healthcare and it happens when she can't speak up or slap you in the head.

When our parents were young and healthy, they were not thinking about the end of their lives. Who does? They based their wishes for healthcare on what little they knew and whatever was written on forms prepared by their lawyers or the medical industry, all the while under the influence, ignorance or apathy of those guiding them at the time of signing. They've guessed, checked boxes and signed documents and now nobody really knows what the person's true wishes are regarding end of life care, not even the patient. All we have is an official looking document that fails in its intended purpose. It only succeeds at being an ambiguous signed document that can be interpreted in many ways.

When we ask people about their wishes for care now and at the end of their life, most say "I don't want to be a vegetable" or something close to it and the rest say, "I don't know" or "I've never thought about it." When it comes to the documents related to healthcare and end of life decisions, very few take the time to understand what they're signing. Most don't care, are nervous, intimidated or simply do not know which questions to ask. Our cultural ADD kicks in, "just as long as I'm not going to be a vegetable..."

Dr. Volandes, in *The Conversation*, tells of a couple who knew each other for 50 years and spent thousands of nights together, shared life's most intimate moments and mundane discussions, but never discussed medical care and end of life choices.[15] In my experience, that's not unusual.

If your medical decisions paperwork came from a lawyer, where is it? I bet you put it in that fire-proof letter box you bought at Wal-Mart. The one with your will, the deed, your grandmother's ring and the title to your car in it (and maybe those pictures you don't want the kids to see). How is it going to provide guidance to anyone helping you with your healthcare when you're old and at the end of your life? Is it what you really want? Do you know what you want? Do you even know what the choices are?

Some of us have more interest, time and perhaps capacity for digesting medical terms and if it's just not your thing, that's fine. Learn what you're comfortable with. After we've taken the first couple big steps toward figuring out our choices (and helping our parents to) we're going to learn about advance care planning visits with primary care providers and how to use them to get questions answered and validate the process.

## DOCUMENT 1

# The Healthcare Advance Directive

It is the bare minimum of what your loved one needs to have in place. There are several variations on the theme, Healthcare Advance Directive, Advance Directive, Healthcare Proxy, Healthcare Power of Attorney, Living Will, and I am sure there are others, but the intent is the same, a properly signed document that names a person to make medical decisions for Dad when he can't and often, in theory, tells everyone what he wants regarding healthcare now and at the end of his life. The person you name to make decisions for you in your healthcare advance directive is called your agent.

There are really only 4 possible choices of what to do when it comes to healthcare advance directives:

**1. Do nothing.**

If you handle things this way and lose the capacity to make your own decisions (even temporarily) you have little or no say in what will happen with your medical care. If you're single, divorced or widowed, you also run the very real risk of having your family going through the ordeal and expense of a formal court proceeding to have someone named as your legal guardian to make medical decisions for you.

**2. Get a healthcare advance directive form from your doctor or hospital, don't bother answering the questions, just leave it all up to the person you name to make the decisions for you when you can't (your agent) and then sign it properly according to the instructions on the form and the laws where you live.**

This path puts the most pressure on the person making decisions for you. They are not sure what you want and you have given them no direction how to make decisions for you. They will be totally unprepared to deal with the medical folks when they need answers and will end up succumbing to the values of family, friends, providers and needs of the insurance company. This is the bare minimum that should be done.

**3.** **Use that same healthcare advance directive form from your doctor or hospital, name an agent, answer the questions as best you can and then sign it properly according to the instructions on the form and the laws where you live.**

If you (or your loved one) are going to be walked through the process with your lawyer when you sign your will or a doctor, nurse or other medical worker when you are sick or old, this is how they will likely handle it. It is cost effective for the medical industry and requires very little effort on your part. My parents just guessed at the answers when they signed their wills. This is what most folks do.

**4.** **Take the time to learn what the issues are behind the questions on the state or hospital forms. Think about them seriously and then talk to your doctor about your choices. Document them in an accepted manner, use the hospital or state forms, with an addendum to express your wishes that are not clearly defined on the form (if needed) and then sign it properly according to the instructions on the form and the laws where you live. Make sure all of your doctors and close family members have a copy.**

Just as there are 4 possible ways to enact a healthcare advance directive, there are 4 solid reasons to take the time to look beyond the preprinted forms and make truly informed decisions about your healthcare now for when you're older and at the end of your life:

**1. Today you can look at the issues with a clear mind. When we have been diagnosed with a serious illness, we tend to panic. By deciding our wishes now we set a baseline for ourselves. We may make changes to our advance directives or ignore them completely in the years to come, but you will have a clear plan in place to compare and perhaps balance your feelings against following a serious diagnosis or even just the realizations that come with the natural aging process.**

**2. Taking the time to make informed choices gives kind and loving direction to your agent. They love you. Regardless of how macho they act, they may well have to make very difficult decisions on your behalf. Doing so will emotionally drain them. It's going to hurt, maybe for some time. The more detailed the direction they have, the easier you'll make it for them.**

**3. It gives clear direction to your doctors. The more detail you express, the less room they have for interpretation.**

**4. It keeps the peace and eases the emotional pain on your family and friends. Making truly informed choices gives them clarity. Just as with your agent and doctors,**

**taking the time to go through the process can negate family members' tendency to project their choices onto you. If you clearly state that you do or don't want a specific type of treatment in a given situation and do so in a properly authenticated and accepted document, there is not much room for discussion.**

Most states have laws governing or suggesting the language of healthcare advance directives. If your state does not, I bet your hospital has a form they like. Some states produce a form all ready to sign. If so, it is probably created by the state hospital association/authority, perhaps in conjunction with a state legal authority.

Lawyers love to write. My legal peers may disagree with me, but experience has taught me that it is better to use the form that the hospital uses than to cut and paste my own. Medical workers, professionals and administrative personnel are not lawyers. They expect to see the same form they ask people to sign. It makes it easy on the intake nurse and the person who has to figure out what it says while Dad is lying on a gurney. Both the preprinted hospital form and the lawyer version should say the same thing because they are based on the same law(s) and/or policies. It's just a different format. If your parents' choices do not fit into the standard check boxes on the form, have a lawyer write an addendum to the healthcare advance directive for you. (Yes, it's ok to question things and to use our own words when expressing our decisions about healthcare.) The addendum should clearly state exactly what Dad's healthcare choices are and your role as the advocate. If you do not like the all encompassing few questions on the state or hospital form, the addendum is where you address those details. An addendum doesn't change the law or the form, but it will make Dad's informed choices clearer.

Regardless of where the document you help Mom and Dad with actually comes from, take the time to have the healthcare advance directive signed properly according to the instructions for the form and laws of your state.

If the healthcare advance directive or equivalent document in your state addresses healthcare and end of life decisions, it probably boils the enormity of the medical complexity down to a few questions about life sustaining treatment (the vegetable question), pain management and maybe something about choices should Mom or Dad have severe dementia. Ask the questions on the standard form to your doctor. Watch his or her head spin with the implications of each one. If they can't quickly spit out a clear yet complete explanation of each question, how is Mom supposed to be able to? This is where the advocate utilizes their knowledge of Mom and Dad in concert with the primary care provider, to make sure that they have the information to make decisions, and that they fully understand what they are signing well before you're in the emergency room with them.

To express our wishes, we have to know the options and neither the prepared forms nor the lawyer drafted ones are going to tell you what they are. Short of having someone in your family with an advanced medical degree who also possesses the needed communication skills, making truly informed decisions regarding one's wishes about medical care seems to be nearly impossible. You need a source of information crafted by medical professionals that is unbiased and tailored to help you and your parents understand enough of the complexity of the treatments available and the related end of life decisions written in language that you understand. The bad news is that the perfect senior and end of life medical care for dummies book has not been written or at least I have not found it. The good news is that some of the information you need has been assembled and it is available, we just have to know where to look.

The science involved with medical treatments is mind boggling. The number of treatments available to us when we are old and at the end of lives does however have a well defined best sellers list. Even if your loved one has an illness that involves the most obscure and specialized areas of medicine, when it comes to end of life choices, there are only so many treatments that the medical folks have to work with. One or more of your body parts is going to stop working at some point and the parts that we hear the most about (I bet they're the ones the medical folks deal with the most) are addressed in three documents, the Healthcare Advance Directive, Do Not Resuscitate Order (DNR) and the Physician Orders for Life Sustaining Treatment (POLST) forms.

We're going to look at 14 questions. Your answers to them will provide the rough notes needed to define and document informed decisions regarding healthcare. The basis for the questions comes from Healthcare Advance Directives, DNR and POLST forms combined with good old common sense. The purpose is to get you and Mom involved in thinking about medical issues beyond the check boxes on the form. Before we're done, her Primary Care Provider (PCP) will be involved in the process. The questions prepare her (and you) for that conversation.

We've been going through this process with clients for a couple of years now and it can be difficult for some. Most want to have made informed choices but don't want to do the work to make them. The reason is that these are loaded questions, no check boxes to fill in with the #2 pencil while watching TV. There are many factors that go into making a truly well thought out answer to each of the questions.

The questions are also difficult because they involve medical issues that we are not familiar with and maybe not remotely interested in. Don't worry, if you don't have a clue, Google it. If you're still not comfortable even making a stab at it, just skip that question. Mom's PCP will help clear things up soon enough. If going through the questions once or twice does nothing more than start the conversion before the two of you get in with the busy doctor you'll be far more prepared to help her make informed choices than she would be otherwise.

After each question you'll see a comment and maybe some humor. That's just to get you thinking. Hopefully, by presenting them this way, you'll find it easier to get engaged with the process. Take your time.

### 1. Would you want to receive medications to relieve pain and suffering and if so, to what extent are you willing to be cognitively impaired?

Raise your hand if you want pain and suffering. Of course you don't. Why the heck would you?

There may be other circumstances in your life that lead you to want the minimum amount of pain medication. I can't see myself wanting any pain, but being impaired (wasted) on pain meds has a down side, I want to know what's going on. You might have a religious, ethical or moral view about it. Perhaps you have many years of 12-step work behind you that leaves you conflicted about pain medicine. Regardless of the choices you make, having your wishes regarding pain relief properly documented makes it easy for you to get what you want and also for your advocate to confidently do their job.

The medical industry and those working in it have at least one perspective too. We read that the insurance companies are spending too much money on our care at the end of our lives and then we hear in the news about the increasing opioid epidemic. I have not read anything about reducing pain medications in end of life situations, but who knows what future cultural pressures will bring. Seeing that your choices are clearly documented provides direction for your medical providers and leverage for your advocate to make sure your wishes regarding pain management are adhered to.

**2. If you have trouble breathing, would you agree to medications, oxygen or medical devices to help you breathe? If you can't breathe, would you be willing to be put on mechanical ventilation (respirator)? If you would consent to being put on a respirator to be able to breathe, are there any circumstances that would alter your choice?**

If something happens and I can't breathe the medical workers are going to want to put me on some sort of breathing machine, most likely a respirator. You've seen them on TV. They may put me on one during a surgical procedure or for any number of reasons. If I am on it for long enough, I will have to be weaned from it and learn to breathe on my own as I am recovering.

Today, at 57 years of age, if it is likely that I will recover from my illness or injury, yes, put me on that breathing machine. My healthcare advance directive clearly states that. If there is any question, then hook me up for a trial period defined by my agent. It also directs my agent to, should I not be able to recover to the point that I can make my own decisions or be able to enjoy a quality of life that my agent knows I would accept, unplug that machine ASAP.

### 3. Do you want the medical treatment providers to attempt resuscitation (CPR) and defibrillation (AED Zap) on you?

If I get hit by some idiot while riding my motorcycle next weekend, and I am lucky enough to have skilled EMTs on the scene when I need them, yes, blue bag me, CPR me, Zap me with the AED and break some ribs trying to bring be back so I can ride again.

When I am 80 years old, have congestive heart failure, COPD, 40% of my kidney function and think that Harley Davidson is the guy in the next hospital bed, I will have a doctor's signed Do Not Resuscitate order in place. If I don't and I have lost the capacity to do so, my healthcare advance directive clearly instructs my agent to sign it for me.

### 4. If your heart was not beating properly would you consent to cardioversion (a medical procedure to restore the rhythm of your heart that involves medication and/or sending electrical shocks to your heart)?

The Mayo Clinic website describes cardioversion as most often being done with a series of electric shocks delivered through electrodes placed on your chest.[16] That sounds reasonable. If my heart gets a little out of tune, fine, tune it up. It gets more complicated when the electrodes on my chest lead to a conversation about pacemakers and implanted defibrillators. Today, if I am told that I need a pacemaker or an implanted defibrillator to give my heart a zap every now and then, I might agree to it.

What about the scenario where I have a device implanted in my chest and it does a really good job of keeping me going, for many years, and I then end up developing some form of dementia and I don't know who my wife is or even when my Depends needs changing? At that point, it makes no sense to have a device in me that's only purpose is to continue my pathetic existence. My healthcare advance directive states that should there be cardiac related devices implanted in me to govern the function of my heart and I am diagnosed with an advanced form of dementia or any other terminal illness that renders me unable to make my own decisions, that my Agent is instructed to have the implanted device(s) turned off.

**5. *If your kidneys start to fail and they want to start you on dialysis treatments to accomplish what your kidneys can no longer do, would you consent to it?***

There are different types of dialysis. Maybe you can do it at home, like a friend of mine did for years before dying from complications following a kidney transplant, or perhaps you have to go to a dialysis center a few times a week, like Janet did. Regardless, your life is going to change dramatically. Dialysis is not a feeding tube, a respirator or an ECU for your heart but, for those who need it, it is life support. Today, with my lack of serious medical conditions, I might start on dialysis. If I don't have, nor will I regain, the capacity to decide for myself, my agent is instructed to not start dialysis treatments.

**6**. *Do you want to be transported to the hospital for life sustaining treatment? If so, would you be willing to be admitted to an intensive care unit (ICU)? If you would not consent to being taken to the hospital for life sustaining treatment or be admitted to an ICU, would you be willing to be transported there if it was needed to keep you comfortable?*

Like most of these questions, we need to answer it in consideration of our medical condition today and in the future. If I am injured tomorrow and the EMTs get to me in time, yes, I want to go to the hospital, very quickly, and into the ICU if need be. Thirty years from now, when I am suffering from a terminal condition or three, my healthcare advance directive will tell my agent to not send me to the hospital under any circumstances unless they just can't do enough to relieve my pain at home.

**7**. *Would you consent to artificially administered fluids/ hydration and medications through an intravenous (IV) line in your arm? If so, how long are you willing to receive artificially administered fluids/hydration?*

Unlike my parents, I know that having an IV does not make me a vegetable. Like all other forms of treatment, my agent is directed that I do not want anything done to senselessly prolong my life and that includes getting an IV in my arm for the sole purpose of keeping me alive.

**8**. *If you can't eat, are you willing to have a feeding tube for artificial nutrition? If so, for how long are you willing to receive artificial nutrition via feeding tube?*

We're not going to try to digest it all here, but there are different types of feeding tubes as well as differences in the content of what they put through the tube and into you. You can research them if you like. I prefer to just look at it in the context of a thick reverse-seared steak on the edge of rare and medium rare, a properly baked potato with too much butter and a good bottle of wine. If I can't enjoy the smell and taste of it, I don't see the point. My agent knows that if a period of tube-feeding will likely lead to my enjoying that bone-in rib eye in the future, I am more than willing to get hooked up.

**9**. *Are there any diseases in your family history that you want to be prepared for?*

The men on my mother's side of the family were shorter than average, round and bald. They smoked, drank and had a good time. If cancer did not get them, heart disease did. My father's side of the family were tall, thin and had full heads of hair at their funerals. They too did what was required to have a good time. They died from the things that come from having high blood pressure and not treating it. I am very aware of my heart, lungs and kidneys, so in my addendum the related treatments get special attention.

If you have watched folks in your family suffer from a hereditary illness, think about what they went through. I'm sure you've heard Mom and Dad talk about how they would do things differently than your grandparents or aunts and uncles.

**10**. *If you have some advanced form of dementia, would that change the way you answered the above questions? If so, how bad would your dementia be for you to change your wishes? Would your age or the nature of your condition(s) alter your choices?*

A diagnosis of dementia, being of advanced age or having one or more terminal conditions will likely change your wishes. The difficult part of thinking about it today is that we want to quantify how and when it will change our quality of life. We have no way of knowing. I've seen folks just answer this with a percentage. They'll just put down 50% or 75% in an effort to give some sort of an answer. If you can't find the words to express your thoughts, just write a short message to your agent and advocate. Don't try to make it sound official. Write what you would say to them, how you would guide them in making decisions for you and tell them that you love them.

You can see from the first 10 questions that age, medical conditions and our relationships to those close to us can guide us to make informed choices. Answering them is hard. You have to think about unpleasant possibilities from not only your perspective but also that of those around you. If you've blown through the first 10 questions and scribbled in yes or no after each one, you're doing it wrong, start over and take your time.

### **11**. *What quality of life are you willing to accept when you're old?*

The first ten questions were foreplay. If you don't put any real time into any of the others, answer this one carefully. Make a list of the things you truly enjoy in life. Then put them in order of reverse priority, the least favorites at the top. As you read down the list you'll come to a point where, if you go any further, you will start to get a sick feeling, maybe you'll just come to that one thing you absolutely do not want to live without or maybe it will be a combination of things. This is not an exact process and you may well change your mind over time. The important thing is that once you've begun to define the joys in life that matter most to you, you are well on your way to giving those that care about you direction regarding the quality of life you're willing to accept and that is far more loving support than most give to their loved ones.

Now for the hard part, write a paragraph or two to your agent and family expressing what you are willing to accept for your advance directive. Don't hesitate to include your list.

If you can't handle answering number 11, that's ok. The other answers will give your agent and family far more direction than the check boxes on the standard form or the lawyers' cut and paste effort.

## 12. Do you want the doctors to tell you the whole truth and nothing but the truth?

Of course you do. If something is wrong with us, we rely on medical professionals to diagnose and treat us. An issue can arise when you realize that they are trained to fix things and sometimes when people die, what we really need is someone who can help control the fall as opposed to catching us.

Doctors are trained from day one to never let a patient lose hope "even when they are obviously dying." Dr. Sherman Nuland won a National Book Award and was Pulitzer Prize finalist for his book, *How We Die*. In it he tells the story of his brother, Harvey Nuland, who he describes as having a "first class mind and two perfectly good ears, not to mention a keen degree of insight." He knew his brother's cancer had spread so far into his body that there was no way he would recover or even live to see the end of the summer. He made the conscious decision to not disclose the true severity of his brother's condition because, in his mind, he could not take away his only hope. By doing so he caused his brother's death to be far worse than necessary. It became obvious to everyone that he was dying. Because of the false hope he enabled, Dr. Nuland watched his intelligent brother refuse logic and all common sense. The "clamor of his wish to live drowned out the pleadings of his wish to know" and that kept him from having any chance at a peaceful death. Telling the whole truth would have hurt immensely but it would have given the family a chance to share in saying goodbye rather than experience his death in a dramatic desensitized panic. Harvey's "...death would have been without the added devastation of futile treatment and the misguided concept of hope." "Almost everyone seems to want to take a chance with the slim statistics. Usually, they suffer for it, they lay waste their last months for it, and they die anyway, having magnified the burdens they and those who love them must carry to the final moments."

What I learned from Dr. Nuland is that even with careful planning, if we're not careful, we might screw up our own deaths. The doctors are trained to never give up hope and most would love to throw that winning touchdown against all odds. Our families are scared and if we don't get our deaths right, it's going to be much harder on them. Our doctors have to know that we don't want any false hope and that our families need to fully understand what is happening.[17]

## 13. Do you want Palliative care?

The California State University Institute of Palliative Care offers this definition: "Palliative care provides those with serious or chronic illness—from the time of diagnosis throughout the course of treatment—care that optimizes the quality of life by anticipating, preventing and managing suffering. It is delivered by an interdisciplinary team of physicians, nurses, social workers, chaplains and other practitioners to address the physical, intellectual, emotional, and spiritual needs of patients and their families."[18]

Palliative medicine is one of the fastest growing disciplines. A good palliative care person can be one of your mom's greatest allies, second only to you. In the hospital, the doctors want to treat every illness and successfully cure it while the administration bills according to the insurance company's payment manual. If the palliative care person has the right people skills, he or she can help balance out the eager surgeon that wants your father with advanced dementia to get a pacemaker or the oncologist that just ordered and is trying to schedule chemotherapy and radiation treatments around his three dialysis treatments every week. If Dad has worked with you to make informed choices about his care, then palliative care, with the right people, can blend seamlessly into what he wants.

At what point would you engage palliative care? This is a bit of a trick question, you can't answer it now. Just being aware of its existence and that palliative care can ease the process for Mom and Dad and also serve as a foil to be used when trying to counteract false hope from being created by overly eager medical folks.

In a way, taking the time to make our informed choices is a type of palliative preschool. If we define the quality of life we are willing to accept when we're old and dying, it will make decisions related to palliative care much clearer when the time comes.

## 14. Where do you want to die?

I had a hospice worker once tell me that she hoped that she would develop a serious form of dementia so that she would not have to suffer the realization that she was dying in a nursing home because she knew her family would dump her in one and not be caring for her at the end.

Many folks tell me that they want to die in their home as opposed to a hospital or long term nursing facility and I could not agree more. Three of our four parents were able to die in their homes, as they wished. My parents died in the same bedroom that they had shared through 60 years of marriage, each on the side they slept on.

Some folks become very adamant about not wanting their loved one to die at home. When asked why, not one has been able to give me a reason other than tears or firm shakes of the head. Maybe they would not want to die at home themselves or perhaps they don't want to taint the memory of the family home with Mom, Dad or a spouse dying there. They may have never talked to their loved one about it and just don't want to deal with death at all. Regardless, they are not the one that's dying.

People close to me have died in hospitals, alone, because a family member spoke loud enough when they couldn't. If you have a preference to die at home, make sure it is clearly expressed in your healthcare advance directive and everyone knows about it. The last thing you need is someone selfishly rerouting you from your bed to a loud and smelly place with way too many strangers scurrying around in the 11th hour.

⌒

The intent of the questions is to create conversation that leads to you, your family and those caring for them knowing what Mom and Dad want regarding their care. I have the following general statement at the start of my addendum:

> To my Agent:
>
> Use your best judgment. Take direction from my Maine Healthcare Advance Directive and this Addendum in concert with the medical knowledge of the providers treating me. When you make healthcare decisions for me, trust in your knowledge of my values and wishes regarding care. You know the quality of life that I am willing to accept. If you think about what I would do, you'll do the right thing.
>
> Thank you for all that you are doing for me.

That statement is far from specific or even close to medical in nature. It is a message that hopefully will give my agent some comfort and direction if they need to make hard choices for me. Your answers to the questions don't need to sound like a doctor or lawyer wrote them.

A person in one of our classes put in their advance directive that they wanted a Viking funeral. Yes, you can do that. You're not getting a Viking funeral, but you will get a laugh from your family. If they're reading your advance directive, they probably need a laugh.

⌒

Once you have all your answers to the questions, regardless how vague and incomplete they may appear to you, it is time to try and fit them into the standardized questions on your states forms. If you can, great, you're almost done. If you can't express your answers on your state or hospital forms, they will have to be expressed somewhere else in the healthcare advance directive. One way is with an addendum to the state or hospital forms. Every question on my Maine Healthcare Advance Directive that cannot be answered in the context of the questions has an asterisk next to it followed by, "**SEE ADDENDUM.**"

For example: here in Maine, our healthcare advance directive gives us the chance to answer 4 questions with yes or no check-boxes. One question about Life Sustaining Treatment in general, one about Life Sustaining Treatment if you have severe dementia and the last two are about Pain Management and Tube Feeding. Following each of them, my healthcare advance directive has "* **SEE ADDENDUM**" in a suitably eye catching font. In the addendum, I have expressed my choices in the context of the 14 questions. The addendum is also typically where you request a Viking funeral.

## The Advance Care Planning Visit

As of January 1, 2016, The Centers for Medicare & Medicaid Services authorized doctors to start billing for a 30 minute advance care planning visit. The purpose of this change in Medicare is to financially encourage doctors to talk about healthcare advance directives with patients and family members.[19] This is significant for our purposes because it provides a terrific forum for us to solidify our parent's choices.

If you schedule the advance care planning visit for the same day as Mom's annual check-up/wellness visit, they can't charge her for two co-pays, so it will save her a few dollars. She can pay for lunch.

If you have been successful learning about the medical terms and discussing them with your loved one, great, now you can get the doctor's blessing at the advance care planning visit and then proceed with signing and sending out copies of the healthcare advance directive and it's addendum (if needed). If you or your father are still confused about the medical choices in the forms, that's fine too. The advance care planning visit is the time to ask those questions and get things cleared up. It does not matter how much of the medical lingo you and Dad have mastered when you sit down with the doctor for the advance care planning visit. What matters is that you took the time to review the forms, are familiar with the some of the terms, made a sincere attempt with the 14 questions and have talked with Dad about it several times.

Doctors are always overworked and constantly being manipulated by financial/insurance related motivators. The advance care planning visit charge to Medicare allows the administrators where Mom's PCP works to bill for the precious time that they should be allotting for her PCP to talk about healthcare advance directives anyway.

The majority of medical folks are not anymore prepared for the conversation than Mom is. This is one of the rare times that having a medical person unsure of what is going on might be a good thing. If you have prepared for the meeting and approach it tactfully and respectfully, the good doctor may look puzzled and even a little miffed at first, but ultimately he or she is going to be happy to have your questions. You will be facilitating the process of documenting her choices. When you go into the meeting, you'll already have a good idea as to what Mom's wishes are. You'll have talked about tube feeding versus IV hydration and the other medical treatments. She'll know far more than my mother did. The doctor will not have to glance at the forms and try to instantly jumble together something that you and Mom can understand. You'll be asking the questions that will lead them through the visit and do so speaking the language of the forms written by his or her peers. Your mother's doctor will be very relieved to find that you've already digested and explained it and should be extremely happy to answer any questions you have and put their blessing on her decisions.

If you go into the meeting with a good idea of Mom's choices, bring an advance directive filled out with a draft of your addendum (if one is needed) for the doctor to review. You have 30 minutes for the appointment. If you're prepared, you won't need it all, even if they have to take a few minutes to review what you've done so far. If for some reason you do go over, you can schedule a second advance care planning visit.

The advance care planning visit adds medical validation to your work as an advocate. When you send these documents to others, be they medical professionals or family members, you can confidently say that you worked through this with Mom and her doctor(s) acknowledges all that has been done.

After you have the medical answers and input from your doctor, and family, then it is time to finalize the form(s) and addendum (if needed) and have it all properly signed. Always use a notary. If the form calls for witnesses but not a notary, use witnesses and a notary. The form has a better chance of working in another state if it is notarized. Even if Mom lives in the middle of Texas, she might spend time visiting others for a month here and there in other states. We want the forms to have the best chance of working wherever she is.

## DOCUMENT 2

# To DNR or Not to DNR,
# That is the Question....

Medical science has progressed to the point that we have machines and techniques (respirators, CPR and AED machines) that can restart our hearts when they stop and breathe for us when we can no longer do it on our own. If you watch enough TV, you quickly come to the conclusion that those paddles they zap you with save everyone. From the 1970's NBC show *Emergency* on, TV doctors have been greasing up the paddles, yelling "clear!" and making folks bounce up off the table so that they can have family members huddled around while unusually attractive medical personnel attend to their healthy selves after the commercial break. That's not reality. The American Heart Association reports that in 2016, 24.8% of adults whose heart stopped, and were resuscitated in a hospital, lived (I don't know for how long). It wasn't broken down by age, but it's a safe bet that the success rate of young athletes is greater than that of 80 year old granddads with congestive heart failure and loss of kidney function. You have less than a 1 in 4 chance of living, if the AED manages to restart your heart.[20]

The law instructs doctors that if there is no DNR in place, they have to try to save you (or at least convince everyone that they are). They can predict with uncanny accuracy Mom's chance of surviving resuscitation efforts. They also know that their efforts can be painful. If you do CPR correctly, you're going to break ribs. The reason they put pads on or grease the AED paddles is to improve conductivity, so they don't sear you too badly.

If your mechanic tells you that your car will be totally rusted out in six months, needs 3K in work to pass inspection today and you should really just scrap it and put the money toward a new one. It is not pleasant news, but it's a no-brainer. You go car shopping. Mechanics and Doctors are human beings, like you. Doctors feel that from their training and experience that they just know intuitively when resuscitation is medically futile on Mom. The doctor may be totally confident that it won't work, but it's Mom we're talking about, not a 280,000 mile Civic, and nobody knows that she will not be of the small percentage that can survive, for at least a little while longer. The problem with you and the doctor trying to decide on a DNR for Mom is that it's her quality of life and rights that you're negotiating. What does she want? It's your job to see that she has the information needed to make an informed decision long before a medical worker comes in to sell the DNR.

*The Journal of General Internal Medicine* published an article entitled, *Hospital Do-Not-Resuscitate Orders: Why They Have Failed and How to Fix Them*. It reached the conclusion that discussions about DNRs frequently don't happen or they happen too late in someone's illness to allow them to make informed decisions. Their fix for the problem is to change hospital culture, reform hospital policies, get the medical workers more training and give them financial incentives.[21] The problems are real, but your Mom is the patient now. The fixes are not going to happen in her (or maybe your) lifetime.

Financial incentives? Yes, they suggest giving the doctors extra money for quality DNR discussions that lead to high ratings on patient satisfaction surveys. How is that different from giving the kid who sold you your last TV an extra $20 for making you see the value in the extended warranty? I doubt that any medical group is spiffing doctors for taking the time to convince a family that Dad needs a DNR and doing such a good job of it that his family takes the time to fill out the customer survey card because they are thrilled about Dad's DNR. I am not trying to sensationalize a wacky idea, I just wanted to interject some sarcastic humor. What the heck, financial incentives might just work. I used to make good money on those extended warranties.

Dr. Brian Goldman wrote of the DNR that "It is a transaction between doctor and patient that is like no other in all of medicine. In almost every other aspect, you see a doctor who proposes a treatment and invites you to consent to it or refuse it. You do not get to demand it." If you do not have a DNR, they are required to try to resuscitate you. You are in effect attempting to force them to perform a treatment and that is not the way things are done. Dr. Goldman further commented that "Most doctors I know would love to be able to decide on their own whether you or your loved one should get resuscitated. In the current system, that's not possible. So we go for the next best thing: *getting the DNR*—that is, subtly persuading patients and families to not demand resuscitation efforts."

Dr. Goldman's words are not offered here to shock you. I value them as a relevant perspective on our end of life choices as they are seen by the medical industry. The motivations behind a doctor's opinion on a DNR for your father are rooted in his training, experience and the medical/business policies of his employers, all under the watchful influence of the insurance industry. If Dad is seriously ill and near the end of his life, the medical folks will come and talk to him (and hopefully you too) about a DNR. According to Dr. Goldman, "the DNR discussion looks like a negotiation. In reality, it's a dance in which we doctors hope to lead patients and their families to see the futility (of further medical efforts) and agree with the doctors." You really don't want a salesperson with a PhD dancing with Dad before the two of you have a handle on his choices. [22]

The DNR choice is not complicated. Either you want to be resuscitated or you don't. It is not the simple question of the DNR that you have to help Dad with, it's the complex and deeply personal issues behind the DNR. The questions really are, do you have a condition or combination of conditions that makes you wonder if you might not want to be resuscitated and what would your quality of life be if you were? Once you help him reconcile those issues, you'll both know if and when he wants a DNR.

The Maine DNR directive form says:

In the event that my heart or breathing stops and I am unable to speak for myself, I, _____ (printed name) direct that no efforts be taken to restart my heart or breathing and the Emergency Medical Services (ambulance crews) if notified, honor my directive. I have come to this decision after considering my condition and prognosis and the potential risks, burdens, and benefits of refusing efforts to start my heart or breathing.[23]

It's that second sentence the makes my head spin, a real can of worms. Essentially, it is a waiver stating that Mom came to the decision of having a DNR on record only after being fully informed and having thought this through completely. If a busy healthcare professional comes walking into the room with a clipboard and a pen for an initial DNR discussion, you better have helped her with the decision long before the door closes and he or she sits down at the side of Mom's bed.

Your job in helping Dad prepare for a DNR discussion is much like it was when you used those 14 questions and your state's healthcare advance directive to help him decide his wishes. You know his conditions, medications and medical history and the two of you have talked several times about his healthcare and end of life choices and then again with his doctor at the Advance Care Planning Visit. You both probably already know the answer to the DNR question.

## Don't Hesitate, Propagate

Now that you've talked with Mom about her choices, been to the advance care planning visit and properly had her sign the advance directive in front of a notary, you need to make sure everyone gets a copy. A copy has to go to each of her providers and servicing hospitals. Just because all of Mom's doctors work for the same parent company, do not assume sending one to the main office is sufficient. It should be, but don't count on it. Send one to every address that you take her to for appointments. In addition, keep a paper copy in your car and have it electronically in your phone.

## Talk About it With Everyone

We've all heard the term dysfunctional family. It makes sense then that if your family is not dysfunctional it must be functional. Sounds to me like the best we can hope for is somewhere around a C- in family functionality.

Your C- family is going to fight when Mom and Dad get sick and again after they die. The fights that happen when Mom and Dad get sick are the worst because Mom and Dad are lying there ringside. Keeping the family informed of what is going on will not make the difficult relatives and friends any more pleasant to deal with, but at least they won't be able to say you didn't tell them what was going on.

You have facilitated Mom's working with her doctor to make choices about her care. If she agrees, you should give a copy to the rest of the immediate family. They may not know the full extent to which the two of you have been working on this. If they have a copy now, there will be less debate about the choices you helped her make when everyone is stressed and in emotional overload.

During the period when you will be the most active as Dad's advocate, everyone goes on a rollercoaster of emotions. The two of you have a slight advantage. You're in it together. That is not to say the process is easy for either of you but other family members often have to add guilt and jealousy to their list of emotions, guilt that they are not doing what you are and jealousy toward the change in your relationship with Dad. We can't control what others feel, but making them a part of the process through communication can cut some of the animosity.

# I Don't Want to Deal with Making Informed Decisions

You've just read a chapter that details a process through which we can make more informed choices about our care. Maybe you, or Mom and Dad, just don't want to bother. Maybe they are at an age where they just can't deal with it. That's ok. They don't have to go through thinking about it, but you do need to make sure that they get some level of healthcare advance directive in place. As for your own healthcare advance directive, now that you know that a method for making more informed decisions exists, if you don't do anything about it, you are making an informed decision to ignore it. All I want is for folks to make informed decisions as opposed to ignorant guesses.

········································

## Chapter Five

# The Rest of the Paper

The heavy preparation is over. Getting the remaining documents in place is going to be far less complex and emotionally draining. Before we get to them, let's take one last look at healthcare documentation.

## *Informed Healthcare Choices as an Estate Planning Tool*

We know that the lawyers and doctors each think the other is helping us plan for our medical care for when we're old, sick and at the end of our lives. The lawyers do not have the medical knowledge nor are they trained to be the complete solution. The vast majority of doctors do not have the time or the training. They think the lawyers are taking care of things because they've been throwing some level of advance directive in with the Wills and Trusts for so long.

Whose job is it? The process that included those 14 questions in the last chapter and the advance care planning appointment you went to with Mom and her doctor resolves the issue of whose job it is. It's yours and you use a lawyer and a doctor to get it done.

Dr. Ira Byock is a strong advocate for and an authority on palliative care. He's an expert in what we go through at the end. In his book, *Dying Well*, he offers a short list of the things most important to us when we think about having a good death:

- **I don't want to die in pain**
- **I don't want to suffer**
- **I don't want to be a burden on my family**
- **I don't want to leave my family with debts or go through our savings**
- **I don't want to die alone**

An effective advocate will use lawyers, doctors and estate/financial planners to dramatically reduce the chances of those fears becoming reality for their parents.[24]

If you've helped Mom and Dad document their informed choices for healthcare at the end of their lives to specifically decide which treatments they want and don't want in the context of not medically extending their lives to unreasonable ends, they have also engaged in a very effective estate planning technique.

## Medicaid and the Egg

We all know that when a person dies their possessions go somewhere. If your loved one led a wonderful life and was either just not fortunate enough, or simply did not see the need, to accumulate what are considered assets by those that label them as such, then, after the Hummels are distributed and you make a few runs to Goodwill, there's not much to worry about. When Mom and Dad's possessions include money, valuables and real estate, they have what I call the *Expectancy Egg*. Expectancy is the lawyer term for what folks think is coming their way as heirs to a future estate, what they are going to inherit. The *Egg* is important to Mom and Dad as well as to anyone expecting a bite of the omelet.

We love Mom and don't want anything from her. It is uncouth to discuss or even think about inheriting things from your parents after they die. Bullshit. Mom wants to leave it to you and you want her to. I don't know how large the estate and financial planning industry is but it's huge, generates a lot of profit for many companies and firms and it is very reliant upon everyone's fascination with the *Egg*.

The *Egg* is by far the most common reason people go to elder law attorneys. Because of our work in the area of healthcare advocacy, we see other reasons that folks call, but, regardless of the stated purpose, everyone is looking to protect the *Egg*. For many, the fear is that the government is going to take it.

The real issue is how to pay for Mom and Dad's care when they can't take care of themselves. It has become standard practice in our society. When we get to the point that we can't take care of ourselves anymore, we move into places of decreasing independence. For a steadily increasing number of us, that means a period of time in an independent senior or assisted living arrangement of some sort before eventually lying in a nursing home bed next to a stranger who hopefully doesn't smell, talk too much or fart louder than our hearing aids' sensitivity level.

Traditional healthcare insurance does not pay for long term senior independent, assisted living or nursing home care which average $5,500.00 a month for an assisted living apartment in Maine to around $10,000.00 for a nursing home (shared room) in 2017 and that's before we talk about the really nice places that we could justify seeing Mom in.[25] Unless your parents have planned well in advance or are more wealthy than most, the *Egg* is going to take a serious hit, if it survives at all.

Some of the confusion and frustration comes from our understanding of Medicare and Medicaid. We work all our lives and pay into Medicare along with Social Security so that we can have a pittance of an income when we retire and access to some healthcare coverage. Medicaid is very different. It is public assistance. Medicaid will not pay for our care if we have any real money to contribute, things to cash in or real estate to sell and it doesn't give a damn about the *Egg*. Medicaid is administered by the individual states and funded by federal and state governments.

Medicare pays for your healthcare, but not the room and board part of the deal when you are in an assisted living or nursing home. If Medicare was ever intended to pay for the room and board along with his medical care, Dad would've had a lot more taken out of his check each week for all those years. When someone does not have the money to pay for the room and board part of assisted or nursing level long term care, they have to apply for Medicaid. If they're poor enough, they'll qualify. If they have too much money, they'll have to spend it down to a level dictated by the state they live in. The law typically allows them to spend it on themselves and their care. Other than in a few special circumstances, they can't give it to you.

Either you or someone from the medical facility that Mom or Dad is going to be in will be compiling all the information, preparing and submitting the Medicaid application. If you're not doing it, you need to either be watching over the shoulder of the person who is or hiring an attorney to keep an eye on things. If you don't know what to be looking for when the nursing home administration is effectively taking over your mother's finances and medical care, talk to an attorney well versed in Medicaid planning.

This has been an extremely simplistic look at Medicaid. There are thousands of pages of federal law, regulations and rules controlling it, and then each state adds a few hundred more pages. You're here to learn about helping Mom and Dad. I've provided just enough of a glimpse to dispel the urban myth that the government is going to take the family home. A more accurate phrase would be that they could very well be forced to sell the family home and give the money along with all their life savings to the medical industry. You hire an elder law lawyer to make sure your parents don't pay any more for their care than they have to under the law.

## Dot and Bill

Dot and Bill lived in southern Maine. He honorably served his country in the Korean War, returned home to work at the Portsmouth Naval Shipyard as a pipefitter, married Dot and raised two sons.

Dot and Bill worked, paid off the house and saved some money in the bank for retirement. They did not consider themselves 'estate planning' type folks. Joint accounts at the local bank were safe and all that regular folks need after all.

Along the way they inherited the family camp. The camp was the summertime center of the immediate and extended family for a period that touched on three centuries. Camp provided Dot and Bill's greatest joy, being with their kids and grandkids most every warm summer day. I never went there, but I can see and smell it.

Dot died suddenly. Bill did not need a house and a camp, so he sold the house and winterized the camp. The excess money went into the bank along with the rest of Dot and his savings. The grieving was hard, but summer came and everyone was back around the fire with a beer or out fishing. Life went on pretty much as we all hope it would. The inevitable tearful eulogizing of Dot on the screen porch, by the fire or out in the boat respected the fact that she died without pain, quickly in her own bed and how lucky she was to go as she did. The family conversation would then flow to remembrances of how others from hers and past generations had died. It became a round of can-you-top-this. Usually those that had lived for years in nursing homes, suffered long cancer treatments and had severe dementia were pitied the most. At 78 years of age, Bill would proudly state, "I'm not going to any damn nursing home, just let me die when I'm old."

One crisp fall day, Bill had a stroke. He was rushed to the local hospital and then transferred to the Maine Medical Center in Portland. It was serious. He never was able to walk again and could only move his right hand a little. He was severely impaired and could not communicate other than smile or cry. He was unable to care for or make decisions for himself. Bill did not have an advance directive, DNR or any other papers to give direction to the family or the doctors. The law does not recognize comments made while drinking beer around a camp fire to be binding choices regarding our healthcare.

A week after the stroke, Bill had a massive heart attack. Because there was not a named agent under an advance directive and no DNR, they performed CPR and used an AED to resuscitate him. After several tries, he stabilized. If he had died then, his wishes would have been realized as best they could have been.

Because there were no documents in place for anyone to manage his care (healthcare advance directive) or his finances (Durable Power of Attorney) the family had to go to a lawyer to have one of the children formally named as Bill's guardian for medical issues and a conservator for his finances. The process involved a hearing (lawyers cost more when they have to go to court), a lot of work for the family in having to gather financial records and fill out a never ending stack of paperwork. They also had the frustrating experience of having to deal with doctors that were not authorized to take direction from them regarding their father's care. A couple months and $20,000.00 later, the kids were in the same place they would have been if Bill had a healthcare advance directive and a correctly utilized Durable Power of Attorney.

Bill needed to be in a nursing home and his insurance from the shipyard did not pay for nursing home care. That meant that his guardian and conservator had to apply for Medicaid to get the nursing home paid for. Medicaid is public assistance. The government will not pay your nursing home bill when you have money (anything more than about $10,000.00 in Maine and as little as $2,500.00 in some states). The family had to spend the vast majority of his and Dot's life savings on nursing home care before Medicaid would pay a penny. Of course the lawyer had already helped them by getting rid of $20,000.00 of it. The camp, because it was Bill's home, did not have to be sold, but most all of Dot and Bill's savings had to go.

When he died two and a half years later, the state's Medicaid recovery folks came looking for all the money that had been paid out through Medicaid for the nursing home. They placed a lien on the camp for the $239,000.00. By this time, there were great-grandkids looking forward to time at the camp. Nobody had the money to pay the bill.

The camp sold for $283,000.00. There were also other expenses, like back taxes and maintenance costs that the kids had to pay on the camp while Bill was in the nursing home, and he had $6,500.00 in funeral costs that had not been planned for. The sons each received $1,860.00 when all was said and done. Forget about the money. One of the greatest uniquely American experiences, the family summer camp in Maine, is not going to be enjoyed by the generations of Dot and Bill's family that will follow.

We have no way of knowing if we are going to die like Dot or like Bill. If Bill had a healthcare advance directive that expressed his informed wishes for care at the end of his life, his agent/advocate would have made sure a DNR was in place immediately after the stroke and he would have been allowed to die when his heart stopped. The camp would still be in the family and there might have even have been a new boat that summer. Dot and Bill worked their entire lives to build something for the family and all they succeeded in doing was feeding a few hundred thousand dollars into the medical industry.

I understand that they did not see the need to plan beyond keeping all the statements from the bank and religiously reconciling the checkbook on the 1st of each month. This is not on them alone. Neither son stepped up to be their healthcare advocate. If they had, and taken the time to help them define their end of life wishes, the great-great grandkids would now know what it feels like to cannonball naked off the float before bedtime (make sure you hit the water with your back). You'd think that Dot's death might have been a clue to someone. Surely the rounds of can-you-top-this miserable death stories around the fire pit should have given someone an idea that they needed to be doing something. There are many variations of Dot and Bill's story that play out in every state annually and all could either have been avoided or at least made less devastating to those involved.

## DOCUMENT 3

## The Durable Power of Attorney

We use the healthcare advance directive to give someone else the power to make medical decisions for us when we can't. We use a Durable Power of Attorney (DPOA) to give someone else the power to make the other decisions for us. It is most often used for financial matters, to grant another the power to transact business on Dad's behalf when he can't or simply when he finds it easier for you to do it for him.

If Dad is a widower, divorced or single and has not planned for his incapacity (he does not have a Durable Power of Attorney) the family will have to ask a court to name and authorize someone to manage his finances for him. Here in Maine, the person named to handle the financial affairs of an individual is called the conservator. The process involves submitting paperwork to the applicable court in your state, usually a hearing (maybe more than one if someone wants to challenge your authority to be the conservator) along with fees paid to the court and even more to your lawyer. Once a court has gone through the process of naming you as the conservator, they are going to want to keep an eye on what you're doing. They will require reporting, usually once a year, which will involve record keeping, your time and, naturally, more fees. Each state has its own laws and procedures controlling how it all works.

A Power of Attorney (POA) and a Durable Power of Attorney (DPOA) are not the same thing. The word durable is important. In order for a POA to be effective when Mom and Dad can't make their own decisions, it has to have language stating that it is *durable,* meaning that you have the power to act for them regardless of whether they have the capacity to do so themselves. The DPOA can be effective the minute they sign it or only when they lack the capacity to make their own decisions. It makes life much simpler if it is effective on the date of signing because that eliminates the need for any debate as to their capacity to make their own decisions when the time comes.

The person giving the power under a DPOA is called the *principal* and the person the power is given to is the *agent.* When your loved one legally grants you the power to be their agent under a DPOA, the law looks at the duty you have to your loved one (the principal) very seriously. The duty is essentially that you owe them your best (a fiduciary duty) and will do nothing under that DPOA that is not in their best interest. That doesn't mean that if your mother can't use her hands and you are the agent named in her DPOA that you can't sign the check if she wants to buy lunch. It does mean that you can't use her debt card to take your paramour to Tahiti, or even buy your spouse a far more conservative gift. If it is not in Mom's best interest, don't do it.

A DPOA ends when the principal who granted it dies. When Dad dies, the DPOA does too, then some combination of his Will, Trust and the laws of your state take over.

Some documents are simply not DIY. It would be very wise to use a lawyer knowledgeable in these matters and I am not saying that because I'm a lawyer. Hiring a lawyer doesn't mean that you are not the most thrifty Google-ninja, master scribe who lives next door to your best friend, the notary. People (especially lawyers) use lawyers for many reasons, including protecting themselves. By using a lawyer to write the documents for Mom and Dad it removes one level of potential question as to your motives and gives the documents that extra level of credibility. Downloading the $19.95 tri-state package from save-a-buck-legal.com is not going to accomplish the same thing.

Financial abuse of our elders is a big problem. Because of it, using a DPOA can be a challenge. Financial and medical folks have to closely scrutinize documents that were once simply checked for signatures and notarizations to be considered good. Most DPOAs are written with no clue as to who wrote it other than the witness and/or notary signatures. Today a notary's mark doesn't always have to be an embossed seal, it can be an ink stamp. People accustom to taking direction from agents are justifiably cautious, sometimes overly so. You should suggest that the attorney write a cover letter that makes it clear to anyone being asked to accept the DPOA that an attorney wrote it and will make themselves available for any questions about the document. Some banks also now have their own DPOA forms that they like. Don't be shocked if you and Dad walk into the bank with your properly written and executed DPOA and the lawyer's signed cover letter to place it on file only to find they have more paper for you.

It can be very frustrating if Mom executed a DPOA years ago naming you as the agent (before she turned 90 and was diagnosed with an advanced form of dementia) if the two of you never presented it to the bank. They may well say the document(s) are too old. DPOAs don't go out of date, but the rules and policies of those being asked to accept and honor them change frequently. If Mom lacks the capacity to sign a new DPOA, you will be calling a lawyer about guardianship for her. Do yourself a favor, get these documents drafted as soon as possible and take her and the documents to the bank (and the financial advisor(s)). Make sure they are on file properly under the policies and procedures of the bank. Test them from time to time. Go in to the bank and transact an item of business for Mom every now and then, just to make sure everything you've put in place actually works.

If the person for whom you are an agent has money with an investment firm(s), take the extra time to make sure the DPOA is properly registered in their system. My experience is that they, more so than local banks, will have specific and seemingly downright bizarre conditions when you use a DPOA. Pack your patience and give them what they ask for. It's far better to deal with a layer or two of corporate mumbo jumbo now than to find out that you can't get the financial records you need when Mom is in the ICU and they are talking about nursing homes.

It is a sad reality that pops up more often than you'd expect. Sometimes, when outsiders see a person caring for their elders, they automatically assume the worst. You and your loved one are engaged in a truly loving and selfless advocacy and caregiving relationship but the assumption by some (often by those who do not care for their own parents) will be that you're only doing it because there is something wrong with you or you're in it for some sort of personal gain. The only gain that matters in our society is money, so the easy conclusion for the troublesome individual will be that you must be after Mom's bank account(s). What sane person takes care of someone else unless there's something in it for them, right? When you are lovingly acting as someone's healthcare advocate others can experience that mixture of guilt and jealousy that can become volatile. All it takes is one person totally ignorant of the true good that you are doing to spout off false assumptions that you're misusing your position as Mom or Dad's advocate for healthcare and agent under the DPOA and it can quickly escalate. As an effective advocate, you are doing a wonderful thing. Cover your selfless butt. Use an attorney to get the DPOA and the healthcare advance directive in place.

## All Fall Down

Aunt Helen was not my aunt. Mom and Helen were best friends for more than 75 years. Helen was older and my mother was wilder (a dangerous combo). Helen did not have any family or friends locally able or willing to advocate for her so I did. At first it was just answering simple questions and as she aged, my role grew into that of a personal assistant and eventually managing her life as her health declined toward death.

Helen was experiencing the early stages of Parkinson's while Mom was in the middle stages of Alzheimer's. They talked on the phone daily got together at least 2 or 3 times a week, bitched and complained about each other and generally acted like an old married couple lacking any semblance of short term memory.

Both had given up driving, which made me their social director and chauffer. They positively loved to be taken out to dinner. No early bird specials for that pair, they wanted to get dressed up and have a reservation of appropriate time at a nice steak house. As their diseases progressed, a better than average steak chain began to suffice, but we never went too early and we always, yes always, had a margarita. I had lunch and breakfast out with each of them frequently because, as you will learn, once you start it, a meal is always a part of the medical appointment.

It had been a month or two since we had gone out to dinner. They read in the paper about a liver and onions special at the nearby steak place and that is one thing I was not ever cooking for them. As the day approached, they started talking about margaritas. I did not respond, hoping it would be forgotten. Fat chance. This presented a dilemma for me. On one hand, I knew they should not be drinking at all and on the other, I do not want anyone telling me what I can and cannot do. On the way to dinner, they were getting psyched for the margarita. I had not weighed in. They sensed my silence was a problem. Sweet and meekly, they asked if I thought it would be ok to have one. I had my position worked out in my head. I was going to tactfully try to dissuade them from imbibing. When I opened my mouth the well scripted argument was nowhere to be found. I simply spit out, "sure, why not" to gleeful giggles.

I had Helen's transport chair (a compact wheel chair with four small wheels) and Mom's four-pronged stick (a cane with four short stubby legs) in the car. They did not want to use them because someone might think they were old. My temporary insanity continued. I agreed to leave the mobility aids in the trunk and go drinking with two 80+ year olds.

With the help of my Dad's expired blue and white placard with the wheel chair on it, I got a spot near the door. Mom's walking was good, but she'd wander if allowed, so I held her hand. Helen was far less steady on her feet and I had to do the interlocking arms thing with her. With one on each side, we made the snail-like entrance that everyone thought was so adorable and were shown to a nice table that Mom and Helen were thrilled with. It was too far from the door for my liking, but, being insane, I didn't say anything.

Before the waitress even handed us the menus, in poor harmony, they squealed "margarita, with salt" and then both looked at me. Why is it that folks engaged in premeditated intoxication insist that everyone around them be on the same bus? I was able to talk my way around a margarita (at that point I really could have used several), only to receive boos and snide remarks from the bad hombres awaiting theirs. They were placated by my nursing a beer.

The salads had not arrived but the margaritas had been slurped up and the salt licked off leaving disgusting lipstick messes on the once stylish glasses. I should never have gone to the bathroom. When I got back, they had fresh drinks. I took a sip of Mom's. They were not the old lady margaritas that I used to make for them back before their medications became unpronounceable. They were not far from what I make at home, when I'm not traveling farther than the kitchen to the couch.

For two ladies with small appetites, they impressively disposed of the liver and onions and wanted the dessert menus. I knew getting back to the car was going to be a challenge and sitting for as long as possible and eating more was a good idea. It was a miracle that they did not think of or have to use the bathroom. With the check paid it was time to head for the car.

Mom went first, almost walking upright, she stayed close to me, fortunately. Helen needed a lot of support which is a tactful way of saying I carried her out to the extent that throwing her over my shoulder was the next method on the list.

Helen could not hear without the most powerful aids known to man. Without them you could literally scream at the back of her head and she could not hear you. She liked to sing very loudly. Imagine Jo Anne Worley at 83, with Parkinson's, buzzed on tequila, laugh-gasping at concert levels. Our exit was not nearly as cute as our entrance.

The drive home was uneventful, just a lot of giggles and the usual repeats of the same stories told whenever the three of us were together.

Helen lived in a senior independent living complex near Mom's house. She had a good apartment as it was one of only a few with a separate outside entrance that could be accessed by a short walk from the parking lot down a slight sloping lawn rather than the walk of at least a hundred yards through the maze of doors and elevators that would surely involve stopping to talk with at least a half dozen of her fellow residents.

I had Mom wait in the car while I walked Helen down to her slider door. We reached the door and I propped her up between the wall and my hip while I unlocked the door. We then made our way into the room and I got her settled in her electric-lift recliner with her walker and transport chair on either side. After she was settled, I headed out the door closing the screen behind me. About 10 feet from the door I heard a loud thud. Helen had decided to walk to the door to wave goodbye, tripped, fell and wacked her head on the pointy ear of a large wooden cat. She was ok, but was bleeding from one of those spots on your head that bleeds a lot. I held the bleeder with a towel and called 911.

While on the phone with the police operator and holding the towel to Helen's head I looked up the hill to see how Mom was doing just in time to see her climbing out of the car. As she starts down the hill to see what is going on, she falls and begins a slow roll down the hill. I was able to get Helen to hold the towel to her head and go retrieve my tumbling mother. After getting her onto Helen's couch, the police and EMTs arrived. Helen was still giggling and Mom was sitting there with grass clippings in her hair sputtering about Helen being clumsy. The EMTs attended to Helen and asked me what had happened. I explained that we had gone to dinner and, knowing the officer could smell alcohol, I fessed up that they had a margarita with dinner. Then Jo Anne Worley yelps out "two margaritas" and begins laughing hysterically. I sheepishly turned my head to the cop, we lock eyes, too many seconds pass and we all start laughing. It makes for a great story today, but I was not very proud of myself at the time. I eventually realized that sour bar mix and ice in a salted glass with two slices of lime passes for a margarita when you're 83.

## DOCUMENT 4
# File of Life

When the EMTs came into Helen's apartment on margarita night, one of them went straight to the kitchen to look on the fridge for the File for Life. [26] It is a brightly colored (usually Red) magnetic folder that, well, goes on the refrigerator door. It contains a form that, if you have assembled the medical records as you should have, it will be a snap for you to fill out. Unless your circumstances are very unique, at some point the loved one you are advocating for will be treated by emergency medical technicians (EMTs) and transported by ambulance. When those first responders show up, they are going to look for a File of Life on the refrigerator door. Check with your doctor, local fire department or police station to find out exactly what they will be looking for.

The only things in the File of Life should be the form your community uses (filled out correctly), copies of your loved ones healthcare advance directive and DNR documents (if they have one) and a current medications list including the non-prescription over the counter ones. Unless your local authorities expressly say it should be included, it does not go in the File of Life. It needs to be updated whenever the information required on it changes (either make copies of the form before filling it in or use a pencil).

The idea is to give them just the basic information they need in an emergency situation. It's not the place to bog them down with all your medical historian knowledge. They don't have the time to learn what you know. The File of Life form, the updated medication list, healthcare advance directive and the presence or lack of a DNR form signed by a doctor tells them what they need to know. Your summaries and all the other documents you've so carefully prepared are safely in your folder (and hopefully your smart phone) and will soon be put to good use at the hospital.

## DOCUMENT 5
## The HIPPA-paper-mess

The Health Insurance Portability and Information Act of 1966 (HIPPA) contains rules intended to standardize and protect the privacy of your medical records.[27] I personally do not care who knows about my 1992 hernia operation or which blood pressure medications I've been on, but HIPPA keeps those secrets from everyone. At times, even from me.

Somewhere there is an underground set of rules regarding customer service in America. They are not openly adopted by management, but every customer service employee that you will ever talk to on the phone or speak to in person has committed them to memory. Rule #1 is to make the person you're talking to go away as soon as possible, at any cost. Not having the right form on file is a very efficient way of getting rid of you, adding to their number of calls for the day or going back to texting, posting to social media or whatever they were doing before you called. To the medical industry, HIPPA is a huge and very costly pain. To the entry level medical employee, it is a gift from the gods themselves, the absolute best way to dispose of you and your annoying questions.

Along with all the other documents you need to put into place, you'll need at least a couple HIPPA releases. The good news is that you don't need a doctor and a lawyer this time. As with all paperwork, do it in advance and use their forms. Ask your loved one's medical and insurance providers for the form they like. After you fill it out and send it in, call to verify that it is adequate and on file, get the confirming person's name and put it in your notes along with a copy and a second original (at the ready for when they claim they can't find it). Don't forget to check the expiration date and renew as necessary.

## Aunt Helen Gets Slammed

Like many older Americans, Helen's insurance consisted of Medicare and a supplemental plan from United Healthcare, sold to her through their affiliation with AARP. When cold called by a salesperson, seniors often do not differentiate between AARP, which provides a nice magazine and the all important discount card from United Healthcare, the insurance company.

Helen loves her mail. She promptly sorts it into piles every morning. One of the piles is of anything related to insurance, medical care and money. It can be advertisements, monthly statements or bills. Anything and everything in that pile requires an immediate call to me, which must be repeatedly dialed every 15 minutes until I call her back and promise to get there ASAP to review, analyze and report on the documents in question. "No Helen, I don't think you need a giant cell phone or that $75.00 pair of reading glasses from the League of Retired Bird Feeders."

Helen called one day and it was not about ads or other useless crap. Helen's entire health insurance plan had been changed. The letter said that she had switched from her two policies to a new one. The new policy eliminated her conventional Medicare and the supplemental plan, rolling them into a single plan managed by United Healthcare. It cost less money each month, so it must be good. I closely read the new and old policies. It did cost a few dollars less, but the coverage was not the same and at that point, it was not the best choice for Helen's particular health issues.

I called United Healthcare and spoke to a representative. I had an authorization signed by Helen on file, so they would speak to me. I asked how this happened and was told that Helen had filled out the forms and sent them in, but if there was an error, we were still comfortably within the time limit to switch back. There is simply no way that Helen opened a letter, read its contents, made a major decision on her healthcare, signed the documents in the correct place and mailed them back without using it as an excuse to summon me for at least one visit. I asked for a supervisor and explained that Helen was of an age where it was very doubtful that she could have done the paperwork on her own and was then told that I must have filled it out for her. Getting steamed, I asked for copies of the new papers she had signed to be emailed or faxed to me and was told they could not do that, but they would be in the mail in the next 14 days.

They never showed and I called several times and spent hours of my life that I will never regain on hold. Eventually, I was told that the papers Helen allegedly signed could not be produced and that they could no longer talk to me because my authorization signed by Helen was now out of date (it has to be renewed annually), they needed a new original signed by her and that one would also have to be mailed to me, in 14 days or so.

Once I was back in the system, I was told that there never was any paperwork signed by Helen authorizing the change. The records showed that she agreed to it when a telemarketer called from United Healthcare. Oh, and by the way, the period to switch back had expired.

Did Helen agree to the change? We'll never know. Someone called a senior with diminished capacity and very bad hearing and told them they could save some money. She might have agreed to it, but even if she did it was far from an informed decision. 83-year old Helen got slammed and it was not just on her long distance carrier or a few bucks to people who take pictures of sick cats and puppies.

Because the new plan was essentially outsourced Medicare processing and it eliminated her supplemental plan, everything from Social Security on through United Healthcare had to be changed back; deductions from her checkbook; direct payments from the bank; my authorization to speak for Helen; and, online access all had to be set up again. Worst of all, to get back where we started from, we had to talk to a telemarketer! I'd conservatively estimate 80-100 hours of time went into correcting the telemarketing switch.

Looking back on it, I shouldn't have asked any questions. Allowing myself to get overly frustrated at the circumstances led me to making an issue out of learning exactly why and how it happened (as if it made any difference). Ego is the natural enemy of the healthcare advocate. Anger got in the way of effective advocacy and even common sense. I should have immediately just switched Helen back when they offered, not bothered to ask how it happened or expended the time and energy.

I have since talked with many seniors who have the new plan and none of them remember how they got it, nor would they have patience (or in most cases, the ability) to make a thorough analysis of its benefits as they relate to their medical conditions or endure the process to switch back. It costs less and they have one bill instead of two. Bless those nice folks at AARP, each and every one.

There was not much that could have been done to prevent Helen being switched back then. I had no clue that it was even possible. The switching time is called open season in insurance terms. It usually happens for two months in the fall of each year. In following years, I had my calendar remind me to check Helen's policy status online weekly for changes during switching season.

## Consent forms

You're probably tired of paper and perhaps a little overwhelmed. That's why I've saved consent forms for last. They involve no preparation beyond what you have done in preparing to be an advocate and require the same skills that you will use in all advocacy efforts. They are also one of the most interesting forms you and Mom are going to be asked to sign, and you will sign a lot of them.

The consent forms I'm referring to are the ones the medical workers make us sign before they do what seems like anything, including an examination or blood work. If Dad goes in for surgery, the surgeon, anesthesiologist and any other doctor that will be treating him is going to ask him to sign one.

Most folks think they have something to do with the doctors not getting sued. Consent forms might find their way into court cases, but that is not why they exist.

We all know about the movements in the 1960s and 70s that helped, at least to some degree, folks whose rights were compromised by issues of race, gender and sexuality. Regardless of how successful you find those efforts to have been, they did create awareness. One area that we never hear about is patient rights, but there was a movement there too. I'm not talking about the patient rights poster so prominently displayed in most hospitals. That poster is propaganda, put there by management, just like the "All Employees Must Wash Hands" sign in the bathrooms of fast food joints. The rights I am referring to are the ones that allow you control over your medical care. As a competent adult, you have a right to refuse medical treatments. You have to know enough about the medical treatment they're proposing (and your conditions) in order to decide whether or not to refuse it, likewise you have to be equally informed in order to consent to it.

The movement for patient rights sought to force the medical industry to take the time with each patient to inform them well enough about the medical treatments being performed on them in the context of their condition(s) to make informed decisions. It succeeded in generating consent forms. In theory, Dad is signing that he has been fully informed about his condition(s), the procedure being proposed (including risks) and that he consents to it. The reality is that they've put a pen in his hand, asked if he has any questions and told him to sign a document that he can't read because they took his glasses, all the while he's wearing a dress with no back to it.

Even in the best case scenario, where all is well and the various medical folks have talked to your loved one about what is happening and they are making an informed decision to go ahead with that heart operation, it's a surgeon and his team doing all the informing.

If Mom plays pickle ball three times a week, goes for long walks, is 70 years old and has no other medical issues and it is within the scope of her documented healthcare choices, the heart surgery may well be the best choice. If Dad is in his 80s, uses a walker, has loss of kidney function and some level of dementia, you and he are very likely to get the same informed sales pitch from the heart surgeon and his team. It is not that Dad's surgeon is necessarily promoting a needless procedure. He or she is trained to make people's hearts work better. They are doing what they are supposed to do, inform you about how they can make Dad's heart work better. Thankfully, you have been through the process of helping him define and document his choices, and more importantly, he has you as his advocate to balance the skilled surgeon's work with the quality of life that he will accept.

## Putting it all together

Katy Butler is a writer and the daughter of a man who ended up with a pacemaker. Her dad was a retired college professor. At age 79 he had a stroke that left him with a fraction of his former physical capability, yet able to fully understand and suffer the frustration of his conditions. A year after the debilitating stroke, he was diagnosed with a heart condition and a pacemaker was implanted. Her parents had not planned for this nor had they imagined the scenario that they would end up living with. In her book, *Knocking on Heaven's Door*, Ms. Butler details what her family went through after they allowed the pacemaker to be implanted in what she calls a "moment of hurry and hope."

Her parents did as they were advised. They planned and prepared just like the medical folks and lawyers tell us to. They had Durable Powers of Attorney and Living Wills written and properly signed. Living Wills are much like the medical decisions portion of most healthcare advance directives. They answered the questions on the pre-printed forms. They did not think about what they would want regarding their own care when the family found themselves in that "moment of hurry and hope." Their planning did not include thinking beyond the forms provided to them and Dad ended up with a pacemaker that "...kept his heart going while doing nothing to prevent his slide into dementia, incontinence, near muteness, misery and helplessness." Ms. Butler stated it well, her parents "had been in control of their lives and did not expect to lose control of their deaths." The documents that Ms. Butler's parents had in place did nothing to provide direction to her in advocating for them nor did they sufficiently express their wishes to those providing care. They trusted that the doctors and lawyers would inform them to the extent needed to make educated treatment decisions and they ended up facilitating business decisions for the medical industry. They did not engage in a process to define and document their healthcare choices and as a result, an 80 year old man, lost his self-respect and was forced into existing with a quality of life that neither he nor his family could bear with no way to correct it, all because they were sold a pacemaker when they were emotionally distraught and lacking the facts needed to make an informed decision.

When Ms. Butler's 77 year old mother could no longer care for her husband at home, they consulted a specialized attorney to learn about paying for her father's long term care. The lawyer was a pioneer in the then new field of elder law, "a ferrety little man in his forties with a straw mustache." I don't think she liked him, but some lawyers are ferrety little men. He told Ms. Butler and her mother that his own father had died of Alzheimer's and his nursing home costs left his family nearly penniless.

The lawyer did what elder law attorneys do. He detailed how Medicaid works and made suggestions about how to preserve assets and other estate planning issues. He updated the healthcare advance directives according the laws of his state using the language of the law without any thought about how it would all actually play out.

Ms. Butler's parents had healthcare advance directives drafted (twice) but they failed to express their healthcare choices wishes for end of life decision making and more importantly, they did not provide any direction for the family. In her words, "We had no idea just how flimsy these paper amulets would turn out to be." How did educated successful folks like Ms. Butler and her parents have this happen to them? I can see where many would jump to the conclusion that this is somehow the fault of the lawyers or the doctors. It's not.

Both lawyers that Ms. Butler's parents went to see, their initial estate planning/family attorney and the elder law specialist, did their jobs. They prepared the correct documents according to the standards of their profession given their training and experience. Every doctor that treated her father did their job as well. The cardiac folks that sold the pacemaker did just what they were supposed to. The heart was not working as it should and they applied the best technology and medical expertise to make it work better. It was not their job to tell them that the heart was going to work long after other things started breaking or to remind them that Dad was old and had already suffered a debilitating stroke. Even if they were lucky enough to have someone take the time and objectively inform them, there were no documents detailing her father's informed choices for care in place to give the family any direction. Lawyers and doctors can't prevent what happened because the nature of their professions and the training they receive simply do not include strategies that account for the circumstances that crushed the Butler family.

Healthcare advocacy is not the practice of law or medicine. We can't outsource common sense. Unless someone steps up as our advocate (or we advocate for ourselves) by seeing that our informed choices for healthcare when we're old, sick and at the end of our lives are properly documented, what happened to the Butler family is quite likely to happen to any of us.[28]

## Chapter Six

How to Advocate, Part I

M edicare and other health insurance providers send Mom and
Dad periodic Explanation of Benefits (EOB) Statements. The
EOB provides a brief summary of recent medical activity that has
been submitted to the insurance company for payment. If there is any
difference between what the medical provider charged and what the
insurance company is going to pay, that amount is shown. The EOB
tells them they might have to pay that remaining balance but several
factors determine whether they do or not. If they have more than one
insurance company the secondary provider may pay some, or all, of
the remaining amount. They may qualify for some form of assistance
program offered by the medical provider. There are also limits as to
how much doctors can charge over the amount paid by Medicare.

Many seniors do not understand the EOB. More than a few of
you just let out an exasperated sigh because you know where I'm
going with this. The EOB says in a large font, right at the top of the

page, *THIS IS NOT A BILL.* Yet somehow, as our parents age they can get extremely worked up over the EOB. They become stressed to the point of sleepless nights, or at least speed-dialing panicked calls to you when the mail comes. It seems that when some seniors read an EOB that the whole *THIS IS NOT A BILL* statement is blocked from their minds by a flash and ensuing mushroom cloud that goes off when their eyes lock on the figures being quoted for their medical care. Logically, they know they do not have to pay what can be thousands of dollars but somehow it scares the crap out of them. I suspect EOB terror is rooted in some aspect of the cognitive decline that is part of the natural aging process, which is even worse if there is some form of dementia involved, but we'll leave that discussion for the experts.

My layperson's common sense tells me that EOB terror is also related to the consumer mentality that we have engrained in us as life-long contributors to our economy. Regardless of our age or cognitive ability we all know that money matters and when we see large dollar values on a piece of paper addressed to us, we get a little nervous. You may not be having the EOB cold-sweats yourself at this point but your consumer mentality needs to be kept in check if you're going to be as effective as possible when working with the medical folks.

We all have our standards. I am not referring to our ethical and moral values. Let's talk about your customer service expectation standard. You expect to be treated in a certain way by anyone remotely connected with the money you contribute to our economy. Whether you're complaining to the entry level customer service representative or the regional vice president, you are confident that you can get that thing you backed your car over replaced for free. Regardless of whether you argue company policy or just mount a verbal attack for reasons justified (or not), you know it's likely that they will eventually give you what you want just to make you go away. Using your ninja consumer skills or just good old screaming will never, ever, work when dealing with the medical industry.

We have seen more than a few patients and family members go ballistic on medical workers and they don't even blink. Most, but not all, of the medical folks caring for your mother are far too professional to allow any harm to come to her just because you behaved like an idiot, but they will remember your actions the next time you ask them for information, or request some less than critical care task be done now as opposed to putting it off for the night shift. They may or may not immediately react to your outburst, but when you're not expecting it, they will get even.

If there ever was an industry that needs to satisfy you as a consumer, medicine is it. Those large numbers on Dad's EOB should damn well entitle him (and you) to special treatment. It doesn't work that way. Dad is not the customer. He's the product. The insurance industry is the customer. Trying to enforce your customer service expectations on Dad's medical providers will be no more effective than the new Maine resident with the house on the ocean demanding that the road he lives on be plowed to remove the snow more frequently than the rest of us because he pays more in property taxes.

You will always be more effective when you calmly work toward the goal of better care for your loved one as opposed to barking at the medical staff. It's ok if the medical workers get mad at you. You just can't get mad at them.

When you vent your frustration excessively, you run the risk of creating a bad impression in the medical workers eyes and possibly affecting your parent's care. When you are calm and the medical folks are not, you have the opportunity to improve your loved one's care. When someone is upset for any reason, you have an opportunity to show compassion and that will make things better every time, on levels you may not even be aware of. You may not be able to fix what has frustrated that doctor or nurse, but your efforts will be ingrained in their mind just as your irrational outburst will be. Just throw it out there, "I can see you're upset, is there anything I can do?" Even if they just shrug you off or blurt out some sharp condescension, you will have changed the energy in Mom's room for the better. If they talk and you listen, communication will happen. You might even make a friend. If that happens, you benefit and, in a most synergistic way, Mom does too. I'm not suggesting that you prostitute yourself for your parent's healthcare or be something you're not, just be the kind participant in our society that you should be and it will all mysteriously work out. You don't even have to chant, sit like a pretzel or sing Kumbaya.

Worst case scenario: you've done all that you should to be prepared, you're the poster child of consistent advocacy (a Jennie clone) and you just feel it coming on. You're overtired, your stress level is off the charts and the level of incompetence you are witnessing is shocking. The new nursing aid is not emptying the bed pans. She's just stacking them in the closet under your mom's clothing (true story). Don't take hostages. Cry. Tears will always work better than foaming at the mouth or climbing into the ring with the security team. You will feel better after a good cry and I've never seen a medical worker who could not be softened with tears. It does work better for wives and daughters. If you can't muster tears, just sit down, sigh and put your head in your hands. Maybe rub your eyes so it looks like you might cry and ask "what would you do if she were your mother?"

The attitude you bring is everything. Even if Mom and Dad wanted nothing to do with talking about care and end of life issues and you have no clue about their medical history, the manner in which you interact with medical workers can improve their care.

I cannot stress enough the importance of listening. Doctors interrupt patients within 18 seconds when they are talking, be prepared for it.[29] You have things you want to say about Mom and her care and the medical workers are moving and talking so fast that you can't get a word in edge wise. Listen to them, be patient, and wait your turn. Listening is not just the crap you have to suffer until you get to talk again. It involves you slowing your head down and being an active participant in the conversation, the one that is not speaking. You also have to be able to hear what is not said. You get that from observing the other person, facial expressions, statements of uncertainty, overly confident statements, talking to fast, talking too slow, not making eye contact with you, staring at the electronic device you can't see, and the attitude they are projecting. *Columbo* would be a great healthcare advocate, Al Pacino's Tony Montana, from *Scarface*, not so much.

From here on in, we're going to assume that you have made a valiant attempt at preparing and you are going to tactfully engage with the medical workers caring for Mom and Dad, leave a minimal body count, and do so confident in the fact that, while you are not a medical professional, you do in fact know much more about your loved one and their medical history than those treating them.

## Yourself

In the safety announcement before takeoff they tell you that if you're traveling with someone and the oxygen masks drop that you should always put yours on first before you help anyone else. Makes sense, if you can't breathe you're not going to be much use to Mom as the plane goes down.

A big challenge lies in balancing your role as an advocate (and most likely caregiver to some extent) with the rest of your life in such a way that you remain at least competent at both.

Jennie's and my father died before we cared for our mothers. Our efforts at advocating and caring for our mothers overlapped. You know the tale of how Jennie used the medical records to help the doctors find Janet's serious heart condition, advocated for her in Boston and then as primary caregiver in her home. My efforts at helping Priscilla were far less dramatic or heroic.

During the time I acted as her advocate and primary caregiver the house was configured as it was when I grew up there. Mom's living space utilized the first floor and the second floor consisted of two rental apartments. She was diagnosed as being in the middle stages of Alzheimer's about the same time that Jennie became involved with her mom's care. When Jennie was spending a lot of time in Boston, one of the apartments opened up in my mom's house. At that time I had finished law school, been admitted to the bar in Massachusetts and was studying for the Maine bar exam while doing work for other lawyers on various projects. Not having a clock to punch, I put Jennie and my belongings into storage and became Mom's new tenant and caregiver.

In advocating and caring for Mom my stress level was always

manageable. Her health declined slowly and she never suffered the horrendous things you hear about Alzheimer's patients and their families going through. She just remembered less and less, slowly forgot how to do the things we learn as children, eventually stopped eating and died peacefully surrounded by her family in the bedroom she had shared with my father for 60 years. We were both very lucky.

It was the bane of our existence as kids, Mom's super human hearing. It was also her biggest challenge as an advanced dementia patient. When she heard something outside, she'd get all giddy thinking someone had come to see her and we were going to have fun. She'd just walk outside without regard for weather, clothing or time of day. It was not a serious problem because I (or a paid caregiver) was always around. Mom was not a danger to herself otherwise. We could not afford 24x7 care and I was not going to park my mother in a nursing home until I had done everything I could to avoid it, so I rigged up a system of a baby video and audio monitors, cow bells and eye hooks with the electronics wired into my stereo system. I spent much of my time upstairs in the apartment studying and doing the law, one eye on the monitors with the speakers turned up to 11. When I heard Mom moving, I'd look to see what she was up to and if the cow bells sounded or the doors rattled under the strain of the eye-hooks, downstairs I'd go. Luckily, I am also a very light sleeper. I have no idea if my cobbled together safety net was anywhere even close to being acceptable by professional healthcare standards, but it worked for us. Mom's doctors as well as the home nursing and hospice folks got a kick out of it. They'd walk in the house and see Mom sitting on the couch watching TV and, having tripped the home-alone alarm system and shown up on the monitors, then hear me come running in. If they did not know about the system, it was unsettling for them to see her alone, knowing that she shouldn't be, and then have me pop out of nowhere.

I was able to arrange for paid caregivers a few hours some days so I could leave for a while and typically manage an overnight every week or two for a visit with Jennie and Janet. Mom's care and the rest of my life were always close to being balanced. It was not memory's fondest 18 months, but I was never stressed to the point that Mom's care suffered or that I lost my mind.

Mom enjoyed the tomato soup that I'd spoon feed her almost every day. It was a favorite and always tasted good to her because she'd forgotten that she just had it 24 hours ago. A grilled cheese, Lobster roll, small piece of beef tenderloin on the grill or Chinese food were other ways of being sure she'd eat. Overall, I'm pretty sure my stress was controlled because I really like tomato soup too.

Jennie's situation was much different. Her mother's care required more of her, at least 90 hours a week and it was in a medical facility, not at home watching Mom on the monitor and waiting for a cow bell. The amount of time and effort was compounded by the fact that Janet was very anxious whenever Jennie was not at her side. That caused Jennie to feel guilty whenever she'd tell Janet that she was not going to be there for a few hours or perhaps a day to come home and visit Deuce (our dog) and I. The self-absorbed guilt, the hours she put in and family stresses sometimes put Jennie in a bad place.

It is easy to argue that if Jennie had taken more time for herself, her personal stress would have been lower which would have benefitted her as well as Janet. On the other hand, Janet had seen time and time again how Jennie caught everything from medication errors to someone forgetting about one of her conditions. Janet was sharp and she knew that without Jennie there, her care would not be as good, she would not be as comfortable and, perhaps most importantly to her, she would be alone and scared. Due to the players involved, it was a difficult one to manage. I can't speak for Jennie, but I would have been more effective if my stress level were lower, even if it meant a little more anxiety for my mother when I was not there. I think most of us need our oxygen masks on before we help someone else, but that is not always possible.

We have to be careful. We're Americans. Justification is our primary religion. Don't use your stress level as an excuse for not being the best advocate than you can. This is going to get uncomfortable. You're supposed to feel it. Nurses are always asking about pain level. "From 1-10, where is your pain?" There is an advocate's stress level scale too. I think my 4-6 stress level with my mom was quite manageable. Mom was a great patient, I did not have to deal with medical workers every day, my family was quite happy leaving me alone in my efforts and I have an unusual amount of patience (got it from Dad). Had her conditions required it, I could have done more. I was fortunate.

Jennie's stress level ran 6-9 most days. I think it was too high, but Jennie has a tremendous capacity for advocating and caregiving. Dr. Brian Goldman gives us a medical slang term for crossing the line into ineffectiveness and possibly hindering Mom's care, *dyscopia*. It is a portmanteau combining dyspnea (difficulty breathing) and dysphagia (difficulty swallowing).[30] I'm confident that you can handle a 5-7 on the advocate/caregiver stress-o-meter without catching dyscopia. Don't endanger Mom's care or your sanity, but don't be a little whiner either.

## Your Loved One

Hopefully, as soon as you bring up becoming your loved one's health-care advocate, they will cry tears of relief and express their undying gratitude, but the odds are that they are going to look at you like you've lost your mind or wonder what you're up to. In Mom and Dad's eyes, we're still the kids. They tell us what to do and we pull the same crap we did as rug rats. I've never seen a working healthcare advocacy relationship that didn't go through some growing pains. In helping Mom and Dad, you will experience all of the stresses that any close working familial relationship produces. If you or your dad is inherently a pain in the ass, that's not going to change.

Regardless of the dynamic, the advocate and the loved one need to work together like a championship team. If that doesn't happen, your efforts will never be as effective as they could have been. It can't be emphasized enough that for you to do the best you can for your loved one, they have to respect, or at least acknowledge and abide to some degree, your role as their advocate and that means not making impactful decisions regarding their care without involving you.

Once you start going to appointments with Dad, you will both see how much better communication with his providers becomes and how much more you both understand about his conditions and treatment plan. At the doctor's office (even the busiest ones) there is a defined list of things that need to be covered during the appointment. It is pretty much you, your loved one, a nurse (or MA) and the doctor working in one of the office's examining rooms for a singular purpose. Nobody hears, listens, comprehends or processes things as clearly while in a hospital as they do in the doctor's office with their daughter sitting next to them.

Unlike the scheduled appointment, the busy doctors, nurses and administrative folks in the hospital or rehabilitation facility are going to ambush him. They'll just pop into the room when he's half asleep, waiting for help getting back from the bathroom or during a tied game at Fenway. It is crucial that Dad not go rogue on you when he is in the hospital. Having the medical historian there for medical consultation and treatment decisions is exponentially more important when he is an inpatient.

Many of the medical workers coming in to Dad's hospital room are working in a vacuum. They are likely doing their assigned tasks with little or no coordination of efforts. If three different doctors order blood work, Dad might have blood drawn three times that morning. When a doctor comes in, he or she has not talked to the other two and may well make decisions without them. Maybe they were too busy or the other two did not enter things into the system correctly. When Dad is in the hospital, being the up to date medical historian is invaluable and it's critical that you be there when decisions are made. If Dad's off making decisions about his care without the benefit of you being there, he's negating a huge part of your efforts.

It will go best if every time a medical person asks a question to Mom (other than her pain level or lunch preference) if she simply states that she would rather wait until you are available to be with her to hear the information before making any decisions. If Mom does that, the medical folks will quickly learn to come with information or ask the big questions only when you are available. If Mom starts answering the questions without you, those same medical folks will also quickly learn that they can get the easy answer they're looking for without having to deal with your irritating time consuming questions. It's less work for the medical workers if you're not there to ask what those other two doctors think about the proposed treatment or medication change.

One of the key factors in Jennie's ability to effectively advocate for Janet was that from day one, they were a team. The emotional drain of caring for a loved one through illness and death is great. Jennie and Janet had the same relationship challenges that they always did and the stress of it all sometimes made things worse. Less than kind words were occasionally spoken and tears shed. What made the team work was the fact that when push came to shove, Janet was respectful, appreciative and supportive of Jennie's efforts. They both held rock solid when it came to presenting a unified front to medical folks. Janet would not make decisions without Jennie.

Janet's greatest love was being with family. Her will to live was firmly rooted in being able to spend time with her children and grandchildren. When Jennie was actively advocating for Janet it meant that Jennie was spending time with her, far more than she had since she lived in the family home as young girl. Regardless of the circumstances, Janet was thrilled to have Jennie around and that made the process of her coming to accept the help of an advocate a seamless one. Sometimes it works like that, but not always.

At first my dad, John, did not want me involved in his care. It was his life and he managed it. He also did not ever want to bother anyone and the idea of my taking 1/2 days off from work to take him to appointments was not acceptable or needed in his mind. We did come to a good working relationship, but I was the one who had to make it happen. Slowly he'd allow me to go to appointments, talk with doctors and take care of the paperwork. I found it best to just talk with him, tactfully guide him with subtle leading questions and support him when he leaned in the direction I thought was the best in the context of his conditions, the current medical opinions and my knowledge of his history and quality of life choices. Far more often than not, it was a battle of patience. His patiently saying no and my patiently asking him the same questions 20 different ways. You need to use the basic negotiation skills you developed when you first started dating. After about 6 months of jousting, he became comfortable having me advocate for him, but I always had to keep things at his speed and assure him that we were managing his care together. He was still in charge, but the dragging of heels slowly turned his morning greeting into a smiling "what do we have today, son?"

An interesting thing happened in all of those conversations about treatments for his various conditions, medical appointments, countless miles spent driving to and from appointments and the required breakfast or lunch that followed. Our relationship changed. We had always gotten along well, never suffering those lifelong father-son pains that many endure. I can't articulate how it happened, but our relationship evolved to a place neither of us knew it could. It was not him teaching me or me trying to assert myself as an adult. It was the first thing that we ever worked on as peers. He was still the dad and me the kid, but helping him manage his care during his slow decline toward and including his death made the whole process easier for both of us. Being real men, we never talked about it, but we were both very comfortable with it all.

⌒

There are some individuals that seemingly can't be helped. They will hinder your efforts at every turn. From what I have seen, they are the rare exception. Most put up some initial resistance, like my dad, and a few immediately embrace your efforts, like Janet did Jennie's. If you do have the rare loved one that borders on insufferable, you will just have to suck it up and do the best you can. So long as the person you are advocating and caring for has not lawyered up and totally excommunicated you from their existence, even the most difficult mom or dad will ultimately receive better care if you are prepared and consistent in spite of them.

⌒

The relationship you have with your loved one is going to be one of the biggest influences on your success as their advocate. I can't tell you how to manage it, but I can tell you that this is not about you. If you can put aside whatever your problems are and check your ego at the door, I'm confident that when all is said and done, whatever it was will not matter and you might just forget a big part of your ego when you leave.

## The Paid Professionals

The process of achieving a license to practice medicine (be it a doctor or a nurse) requires a superhuman effort. The vast majority of us could never do it. Those that succeed to the point of getting a prescription pad deserve your respect, at least until they conclusively prove to you otherwise.

The commitment of time and money along with the level of discipline required to become a doctor is much greater than any other profession that I know of. If you undertake what is required, most of you will not be attending the school you wanted (if accepted at all), will be graduating in the middle of your class and there is absolutely no way you will be working at anything close to the rewarding job you envisioned. Becoming a leading medical professional is about as likely as becoming the next NBA superstar.

As you interact with doctors, please remember that my efforts here are to help prepare you to be Mom and Dad's advocate. It is not my intent to belittle the immense amount of work that is needed to become even a below average doctor or nurse. I admit to trying to demystify and humanize the industry for you but do not let my attempts at dry and often sarcastic humor taint the profession of medicine in your mind.

When I was a middle-aged man thinking about going to law school, I bought a book entitled *Law School Confidential* by Robert H. Miller and a team of others. The target audience was not middle-aged folks, but it did provide some insight to the brain scramble that I was about to pay good money for. Mr. Miller wrote another book with a different team of folks, *Med School Confidential, A Complete Guide to the Medical Experience, By Students, for Students*. It popped up on Amazon one day. I added it to the cart because that is what we do when things pop up on Amazon. I did not expect any great insights on healthcare advocacy, but it is interesting how portions of it echo the words of medical industry commentators.

The forward was written by Harold M. Friedman, MD. He was,

at the time of publication, a professor and the Chair of the Admissions Committee at Dartmouth Medical School. In a book aimed at young people thinking about medical school he addresses the things we would expect such as ethics, concern for patients as individuals, diversity in education to enrich your life and so on. He also wrote:

> You have an obligation to try to be certain the new technology or drugs are cost-effective, not just something new with marginal benefits. Cost containment and rigid practice guidelines, when based on good clinical data, may save resources of both society and your patient. Everything you do must be tempered by the notion that your first obligation is to your patient and not to enhance your own income, the groups, or an insurance company's.[31]

If I am a young person trying to pick my undergraduate major with an eye to possible med school or a recent college grad with my science degree in hand, I would (had I bothered to read the forward) find that paragraph odd and maybe even puzzling. I'd expect to be advised to not make personal gain the only reason for picking any career, but other than that, the rest of it comes from way out in left field. Dr. Friedman was 71 years old when the book was published. When he wrote those words to that young audience, he had witnessed tremendous changes in the science and business of medicine. Regardless of whether or not he approved of those changes, he made a clear point to those considering a career in medicine that business controls the care provided. When stating that the doctor's first obligation is to his patients, it is not done in a standalone sentence. He tempers the point by telling us the challenge to a patient being a doctor's first priority is greed, personal, and that of their employers and the insurance companies.

⁓

Medical students get two years of time in the classroom and then two years that are sort of an apprentice period where they work in different areas of medicine, each for several weeks at a time. They are interacting with patients, but not making serious treatment decisions yet. The students do patient intake interviews and when they have proven themselves they are allowed to do some patient examinations. Of examinations, our prospective medical students are told that they will see the more experienced doctors "cutting corners and hitting only the high points of an exam, but at this stage you should err on the side of being more thorough."[32] That's right, our future doctors, only a few pages after being told that they need to follow rigid practice guidelines, are informed that it is ok to only hit the high points of a patient's examination, it's just that they should not start doing it too soon. They have not even applied to med school or in some cases graduated high school and the kids thinking about being our healthcare providers when we're Mom and Dad's age are already being told it's ok to cut corners and that business is more important than medicine.

Dr. Jerome Groopman tells us that "medical students and resident doctors are being taught to follow preset algorithms and practice guidelines in the form of decisions trees." He goes on to comment that the next generation of doctors is "being conditioned to function like a well-programmed computer that operates within a strictly binary framework."[33] As I understand it, the complexity of the science involved today combined with the economic pressure on doctors and medical students is so overwhelming that they need help to diagnose patients more efficiently. The help comes in two forms, algorithms and practice guidelines. Dr. Groopman noted that the insurance companies like this system because it saves time and money. Independent and creative thinking takes longer and is never cost effective.

The algorithms look to me like 1980s management flow charts. I am sure that I could never understand the algorithm sheets (there must be an app now) but imagine blocks on a page, at the top is the patient with a headache. Below that are two blocks one is marked "nothing else wrong, go to step three" and step three says "take two aspirin and call me in the morning." The other block on the second branch of the tree splits off into things like vomiting, other symptoms and it goes on to help the doctor or student figure out what is wrong with you. The algorithms cannot account for the corners that may have been cut during Dad's examination.

Practice guidelines were also mentioned by Dr. Groopman. They are more of a summary of how a condition is treated by doctors, the currently accepted practice for a given condition or treatment. The U. S. Department of Health and Human Services, Agency for Healthcare Research and Quality maintains the National Guideline Clearinghouse which has a website with public access.[34] If you're not comfortable reading medical material that is way over your head, I'd advise not looking into the guidelines. If you view such things as a foreign language puzzle to be transcribed into English, knock yourself out. Be warned, it takes 8+ years of specialized education to speak Guideline fluently.

Sir William Osler is a giant in the history of medical education. His writing influences every doctor practicing and in training. He pretty much invented the medical residency. Having the majority of his career in the 1800s, students today might see him as outdated and irrelevant to the modern science of medicine. They can Google their way around Olser, but he still impacts the way they will act when treating Mom and Dad. One of his famous works is an essay entitled, Aequanimitas, which loosely means even or calm mind. In it he gives direction to young doctors about the image they should project to insure control of the relationship and instill patient confidence. His essay uses the dense language you'd expect from an academic rock star from the 1800s, but his message to doctors is to never, ever, let them see you sweat. Doctors today call it detachment.[35] The idea is that if you do anything other than project that you are the know all, be all, you will be less of a doctor because a real doctor never lets a patients see "the slightest alteration, expressive of anxiety, or fear" because they are "liable to disaster at any moment."[36]

Even if this is not taught rigorously, only casually mentioned or even joked about in modern medical education, the idea of never letting your patients see anything less than a confident and detached attitude is ingrained in every doctor you will encounter. Hopefully, they will make an effort to communicate effectively, but, they have been trained in and do keep at the ready, that attitude. At their discretion, they can give you anything from detached to cocky. When you are advocating for Mom and Dad you are trying to communicate with someone possessing a doctorate level poker face that has been honed to perfection.

⁓

When you ask a lawyer a question, the answer will typically start with some variation of "well, it depends..." followed by a long explanation that irritates you. That is because you have asked what seems like a perfectly reasonable yes or no question, but in reality, within the law, it involves many variables and there is no quick and easy answer. Unless you are willing to be patient and take the time to understand the answer and the lawyer has the skill to effectively communicate with you, it's going to be a frustrating experience for both of you. The same thing happens when talking to Dad's doctor, but they are not typically skilled or trained at interpersonal communication and even if they were, it was likely the equivalent of optional gym class in med school.[37] To some extent, they are conditioned to believe that you can't possibly understand the answer.

To a doctor, the answer to your simple question about Mom's treatment plan can have several correct answers and they all involve big-bang level science tempered by their clinical experience, all filtered through the medical, hospital, legal and insurance powers that oversee what they do. Before you have finished asking your question, a doctor's mind is generating at least one answer that includes very few words that you can pronounce. When you add the complexity of the doctor's work load, the odds of you getting a respectful answer that you understand drop considerably. It's not just doctors and lawyers. The same thing happens to me when I talk to IT folks or millennial beer geeks.

## The Hamster Wheel

Dr. von Trapp always put the patient first. She was Jennie's doctor and eventually mine. After working for several family practice groups she opened her own practice at a time when that just wasn't done. When I asked why she went out on her own, she explained that working for a group is like being on a hamster wheel. You just keep spinning and not getting anywhere. She did not have the time she wanted to spend with patients so she opened her own office.

By being able to take the time she needed she was able to very effectively treat Jennie after a bad car accident. Before Dr. von Trapp, Jennie suffered from a complex illness that took her through many doctors from southern Maine to Boston. They played pharmacy roulette with every drug they could think of without any consistent success. Dr. von Trapp had the time to work out in the fringes, to do some research, and she was able to improve Jennie's quality of life substantially. By getting off the hamster wheel, she was able to be a better doctor for Jennie.

Unfortunately, there is no happy ending to the tale of Dr. von Trapp. It turned out that the only reason that her practice was able to exist was by operating at a huge loss every year. The insurance portion of the medical universe would not pay for her to run free-range, off the wheel. The whole operation was afloat because of her husband's successful business. When it failed, her practice had to close.

Theresa Brown has a PhD in English, taught for three years at Tufts University and then decided to go back to school to be a nurse. She wrote a book, *Critical Care*, about her experiences as a new nurse. Her book also popped up on Amazon and because Garrison Keillor said that English majors are cool, I put it in the cart.

Ms. Brown writes well about the tremendous amount of work piled onto nurses by the medical industry. The enormity of what needs to be done in one shift often cannot be completed. She describes the strategies used to push work off to the next shift. It makes perfect sense. If you can't get to it all before your work day is done, put out the fires and stick the next person coming in with the rest of it. Unfortunately, there is no way for us to tell what is deemed to be unimportant. Is it just data entry, doing an intake on Dad who has been lying in the ER for two and half hours or is it responding to Mom's call button? Ms. Brown tells us that nurses are trained to prioritize patients, "even the most novice nurse thinks about patients in terms of a need hierarchy" and that she ranked her "patients in terms of least potentially work-intensive to most." I gather from the context that work-intensive can mean medically demanding or just demanding of a nurses' time.

Patients that are demanding of a nurses' time quickly end up like the little boy who cried wolf. They have ways of dealing with painful patients and also juggling too many patients. One technique mentioned in the book is to tell the patient, regardless of the question, "let me check" and checking can take as long as they like. It's not hard to see that the patient end of patient management can be a very frustrating experience.[38]

George Carlin is often credited with saying that "Most people work just hard enough not to get fired and get paid just enough money not to quit."[39] To the medical industry, I'm an outsider, a layperson. When writing about the medical workers, I have to rely on my observations which are tempered by the written words of industry insiders and my 40+ years in the workforce as an employee and employer. Regardless of education, compensation, age, or experience, your effectiveness and satisfaction as an employee is most influenced by how you were trained, the work ethic (or lack of) that has been instilled in you, the culture your employer thinks they have fostered and the degree to which you buy into it.

## Work Ethic and Culture

Mary was one of Janet's in-home caregivers. She was unique in that she was a young woman that could relate to older patients. She took the time and had the patience to communicate on their wavelength, a kind, mature soul in a young woman's body.

Like several of Janet's caregivers, Jennie remains in contact with Mary, so we get to follow her career in medicine. Private home caregivers do not make a lot of money and most receive few (if any) benefits. If they work through a service it is probably minimum wage and overpriced health insurance. Mary decided the best way to move up would be to work for one of the area hospitals. She needed to be a certified nursing assistant (CNA) for which she attended a local college. In addition to working well with older folks, she is highly intelligent and possesses an unusually strong work ethic. She polished off the needed class work in about 1/3 the usual time that it takes. Her internship lead to an entry level job with a home care group owned by one of our better local hospitals. She was making slightly over minimum wage, had benefits, a boss that was thrilled to have her and Mary was feeling good about life overall. Her first job was giving baths to homebound patients, 8-12 in a day. Imagine it. You get up earlier than the 9-to-5 crowd, drive your own car around the local towns, give 8-12 handicapped and disabled folks a bath/shower in their homes and if you're lucky, get home when the 9-to-5ers do. If you're Mary, it goes well for more than a year. Her great outlook, personality and ability to be the grandparent whisperer combined to make the experience as good as possible for the patients and rewarding for her. Even super woman can only give 8-12 baths a day for so long without losing her mind. Fortunately, the local hospital saw far more in her than 8-12 baths a day and moved her into the hospital doing work that provides a better value for them and is also varied and more rewarding for Mary.

Mary got out in time, but how long do you think it takes for those with less of a work ethic or kind heart to seriously develop a bad attitude after a year of giving 8-12 baths a day? How do you think the conversations go when several disgruntled bath givers go out for drinks after work? It is not any different than any group of co-workers that go out for drinks. They complain about work. It can be a simple healthy vent session or it can become a festering downward spiral that drags the positive folks along with them. It does not take long to engulf an organization by creating a toxic work atmosphere that can drive great workers like Mary out the door or break their spirit and pummel them into mediocrity.

Dr. Brian Goldman's book, "The Secret Language of Doctors" provides insight into the slang used by medical professionals. I thought a book about medical slang might be fun to read but ended up being alternately entertained and appalled by what I read. The humor stops when you realize the negative affect it can have on Mom and Dad's care. Yes, it is healthy to have fun at work, but when the humor is rooted in a deep frustration with your work, it becomes a conduit to a seriously bad work ethic. It can destroy the culture of an organization.

In my experience, when someone is unhappy at work, their attitude usually spirals downward to the point of uselessness and eventually they become a hindrance. Management experts have a term for broken employees, *disengaged*. According to the Gallup folks the odds are better than 50-50 that the medical worker taking care of

Mom and Dad is disengaged to some measurable extent. They also report that the number climbs to better than 70-30 if the worker is a millennial.[40]

Jim Haudan is an expert on broken employees. In his book, *The Art of Engagement*, he dedicates one chapter to each of 6 reasons why employees are not engaged with their work:

> *I can't be engaged if I'm overwhelmed.*
>
> *I can't be engaged if I don't get it.*
>
> *I can't be engaged if I'm scared.*
>
> *I can't be engaged if I don't see the big picture.*
>
> *I can't be engaged if it's not mine.*
>
> *I can't be engaged if my leaders don't face reality*

We could write pages about how each of those 6 reasons can lead to poor care for Mom and Dad but that is for the experts like Mr. Haudan to apply to the medical industry. He uses simple language, analogy and humor to make the complicated behavioral concepts understandable to folks like us.

In discussing why workers can't be engaged if they are overwhelmed, he uses the example of Taco Bell. They were sending out so many policies, orders and instructions to the restaurants that the employees could not keep track of them all. There were not enough hours in the work day to read, learn and implement the changes. To show how all of this bogs down organizations Mr. Haudan uses the most sophisticated of management tools, the whack-a-mole diagram. He takes the plethora of usually conflicting policies and edicts and sketches them out like the kids game. I bet if Mr. Haudan took a look at Janet's local hospital he could draw one heck of a whack-a-mole diagram.

The Three Mile Island disaster is also used as an example. The investigation that followed the worst nuclear accident in US history did not find that the control room operators made mistakes. They found the fault to lie in the design of the control room. The next time a nurse or a doctor gives you some attitude or makes a mistake, remember that they may not be the real problem with Mom's care. [41]

## Single Point of Contact

Dad is loved by many. Family and friends want to know what is happening with his care immediately and they will have many stories of similar medical events that have happened to them or others that need to be shared. They'll feel a need to talk to the doctor and nurses themselves and offer their stories. This is a huge waste of time for the folks taking care of Dad. For that reason, most inpatient medical facilities want to establish a single point of contact with a patient's family. Clearly, you need to be that point of contact, but that leaves you to be the one relaying everything to the masses and hearing for the 18th time about how Uncle Louie had a stroke and then fell and broke a hip while having a bunion worked on at the podiatrist's office. You only have so many hours in a day to advocate for Dad and do not have time to update everyone and hear all the stories. You can't win, but you can cut your losses. Being the advocate and single point of contact does not make you the on-demand press secretary.

There are two types of folks you'll be dealing with, connected and not. If there are members of your family or friends who do not use computers, appoint a deputy. You know who it is. It's that one family member or friend that is always at the epicenter, the hub of the news (*news* is what my mom and grandmother called gossip). If you call them with an update or have someone print out your update emails they will be happy to be the press secretary for the unconnected.

Email is better than texting or social media. Texting is too short of a leash. If you send a text to several people, it becomes a conversation. You get hooked into it because they know you have your phone handy. You don't have time for that and it appears rude if you stop responding. I don't mind being rude, but the problem is that they get mad and start calling incessantly. It is less fun, but overall it's better to not be rude.

I do not actively participate in social media. I get it, I just don't have the time. My issue with social media as a way to communicate about Dad's condition is that it is too public. People feel a need to post things that they would never say in person. You don't need that. Some folks feel the need to post every painful detail of their life experiences. Mom and Dad would not want you broadcasting about how they're going into hospice care makes you feel about that incident at your 16th birthday party.

Email works great. You can compose it over several hours or even days, there is no rush, folks do not expect an instant response (they know you're busy taking care of Dad) and you can keep it from becoming a conversation, just don't reply to the silly responses and questions stemming from your update emails if you don't have the time. For some reason it has become acceptable to not respond immediately to personal emails.

Your emails need to be updates as opposed to play-by-play reporting. If you send an email to a group about something that has not happened, you're going to get replies, calls and texts about what you should be doing. Nobody has done the work that you have nor are they engaged in Dad's care like you are. That will not prevent them from ignorantly telling you what to do or what happened to Uncle Louie. If you send the email after the medical decision has been made, or the event has happened, others tend to not feel as compelled to be armchair quarterbacks. Telling the extended family and friends that Dad is thinking about getting a pacemaker is NOT what you want to do. Tell those that need to know before, but release it to the masses after he decides.

## Bed 809B

I have an unhealthy attachment for my old man truck. When it's down at the corner garage and its slot on the greasy blotter calendar comes up, I am sure that they don't say "please drive Mike Guy's truck in and put it up on the hydraulic lift." They say "get that 94 Chevy" or something more colorful. Your Mom is a person, but she is 809B to most of those caring for her.

The organizations caring for Mom and Dad may have hundreds of employees, but if you are lucky enough to see the same ones regularly, know their names. Even if they never learn your name or your dad's, it makes a difference that you know theirs. It's not just the doctors, you need to know the names of the nurses, CNAs and the folks that work at the desk. Do not forget the non-medical workers. The quiet folks that clean and do maintenance work are also eyes and ears. They rarely get spoken to and are often treated as scullery. If you learn their names and are kind, good things will happen. Not the least of which is that they too will have a greater awareness of your mother. They won't be treating her, but will be able to tell someone when she needs help.

When your parents are inpatients there will be at least two or three shifts of individuals working on the floor and some fill-in folks as well. If you see an unknown face in Dad's room, introduce yourself and after they have left, write the name down along with what their job is before you forget.

Knowing someone's name is a sign of respect and it also puts everyone on notice that you are engaged in this process. The more that you do to create a positive mental connection between the person in bed 809B (Mom) and you the better off she'll be. The name connection leads to a greater awareness of your loved one as a person, and that directly translates to better care. They're all numbers, but Janet is Janet. If they never learn your name, that's fine. The fact that you know theirs will still create the connection. When I'd walk onto the floor in Boston to see Jennie and Janet and the staff would just tell me where they were in the building without having to ask or introduce myself, they didn't know my name. They did make the connection between Janet, Jennie and I. When that happens, you know the staff is engaged in Mom's care beyond wondering if there's anything still to do in 809B.

⟋

If you have a medical professional in the family or in your circle of friends, leverage them. Most medical folks love to talk about what they do because their friends and family are sick and tired of hearing about troublesome patients and coworkers. If you can get a dialogue going with the occasional call, email or text, that person will become invaluable. Jennie's cousin Anne has been a nurse for several decades. She became a wonderful source of insider information as well as sounding board for her and Janet.

One thing that Anne suggested was to put a picture up of Janet when she was a healthy active woman doing something she loves as opposed to just being 809B. Jennie put up an 8x10 of Janet in a pool with a dolphin. The effect was amazing. The staff quickly connected Janet with the woman smiling on a warm sunny day hugging Flipper. The dolphin was important. The photo should have other elements in it that create connections and conversation. Many of the most angelic medical workers are not outgoing conversationalists, all they need is a way to engage. A high school photo from 1940 will not create a lot of conversation. Everyone loves animals. Connect Mom with the medical workers through images of her having fun doing cool things.

Jennie noticed that as the shifts changed and folks came and went that many did not have or take the time to read the little details in the chart. Jennie took Anne's photo idea further and put signs up.

Janet had a device in her left arm called a fistula. It allows for connection to the dialysis machines. It is surgically implanted and needs to be protected and if not, it required a three hour surgery to repair or replace it. They were not supposed to draw blood from the left arm, but the medical workers never remembered. Jennie bought a stack of bright neon, multicolored paper and made a sign. "*NO LEFT ARM BLOOD DRAWS.*"

Due to the very low level platelets in her blood, when Janet bled, she bled a lot. When you are on and being weaned from a respirator, they have to suction fluid from down in the throat from time to time. If they went too deep on Janet, she would bleed and that was a serious problem. The next sign, in a different bright color, said, *"NO DEEP SUCTIONING."*

Another sign, posted behind Janet so she could not easily see it, said *"IF PATIENT GETS FORGETFUL, CONFUSED OR SAD, PLEASE CALL JENNIE @ (207-xxx-xxx) TO COME SIT WITH HER."*

Janet wanted to know what was being done to her at all times so yet another sign of a still different color said *"PATIENT REQUESTS TO BE AWAKENED AND INFORMED WHEN MEDS (VIA IV) ARE GIVEN."*

The signs received mixed reviews from the staff and family. At first the signs were torn down or modified to insult and offend Jennie. After the initial adjustment period, they were allowed to stay. In one facility, there was a battle over them. The staff wanted them down and Jennie asked why. Lacking a reasonable explanation, the issue worked its way up the chain of command and seemed to stall one level up from the floor. Around that time, a visiting executive from the corporate owners of the facility happened to be on the floor, saw them and commented, "that's a great idea, when did we start doing that?" The signs were not an issue from then on.

During one of our healthcare advocacy classes a woman who happened to be a case manager at a local hospital also mentioned what a great idea it was and how she wished the staff where she worked could put up the signs themselves. They can't because of the HIPPA privacy rules. The staff can't put them up, but you can. (Of course, Jennie would ask permission first).

# Chapter Seven

........................................

# How to Advocate, Part II

## Too Much is Not Enough

It's rare, but once in a while, doing things the easy way is better. For many, were their Mom in a coma as Janet was at first, they'd go home, brew a pot of coffee or uncork a bottle of wine and then open a half dozen Google windows. Some might just look up platelets, comas, heart valve replacements and print out a few pages. Others would dig deeper. They'd put real time in to it and look up possible drug interactions between her older medications and the new ones. Some will look up the disease or condition(s) on the doc.coms to learn about the likely progression, treatments and prognosis for their loved one. It starts out as innocent curiosity but becomes a problem when we begin to think that our caffeinated or buzzed hours on the internet qualify us to have in-depth discussions or treatment debates with Mom and Dad's doctors.

Dr. Brian Goldman refers to a layperson's internet research as "Dr. Google."[42] He points out that when laypeople go to Google they often only find a part of the information needed to make medical decisions. He is a tactful professional and did not come out and say it, but we only take Google as far as needed to say we "looked it up" or to get the answer we want, good or bad, right or wrong.

Dr. Goldman does not dislike Google. He thinks folks should use it to "get engaged in their own disease management" (or that of our parents). I take that to mean that the internet is useful as a tool to help us understand what the medical workers tell us and to define the big words that we hear and read in the records.

Other than as a dictionary or condensed encyclopedia, Google is not an efficient use of your healthcare advocacy time. The vast majority of what you find will be unreliable internet crap put there to lure you to a place where either you give them money or, yet again, become a data mining statistic. Even if you had a couple years of pre-med or nursing school and have Googled the correct information, trying to play doctor is still a mistake. You don't have the knowledge, medical data, skill or clinical experience to correctly interpret what you're reading and acting like you do will get a reaction from Mom's doctor somewhere between irritated and insulted, guaranteed.

Playing doctor is the hard way and will rarely work. Even if you're correct and somehow force the medical folks to acknowledge it, you will have won a battle but at what cost? You're much better off working with the doctor as opposed to trying to convince her or him you are their peer.

## Ask questions

We know that doctors follow flow-charts (algorithms) and guidelines. When the equation is solved, move on. Next patient please. In *How Doctors Think*, Dr. Groopman tells the story of a man who comes into the ER to have his leg x-rayed after a fall. They assured him it was not broken and he happily went on his way. Nobody asked how or why he fell. It was later learned he had undiagnosed anemia. Dr. Groopman goes on to state that patients do not remember "key aspects of their past medical history."[43] The man who fell may have had other things in his history or even current symptoms that would have provided clues to the ER folks but either he did not remember them or did not deem them important. In his mind, he fell and hurt his leg, end of story.

You will also find that the busy medical workers often do not have the time to listen to the history of an older person. If Dad has three specialized conditions and the doctor treating him for the fall concludes they are not important to the treatment being given, listening to Dad is going to take more time than his or her busy day will allow for. The clues related to other possible conditions are not coming out.

If the patient does not offer more information, they do not have an effective advocate or the doctor does not have the time to ask probing questions, what happens? Dad gets x-rayed, sent home and they don't find the anemia. That must be the doctor's fault, right? No, it's not. It's just the business of medicine. The hamster wheel runs at a steadily increasing speed and that keeps the medical folks from having the time to look closely at a patient and ask *I wonder if*. Medical professionals are trained to look deeper, to ask leading questions that will uncover more about a patient that will lead to better care, but the business of medicine does not allow even the most well trained and talented doctors and nurses to be the best they can be. That's why we have to know which questions to ask and when to ask them.

When we look at the positive relationships that Jennie was able to build with the various medical professionals at the local hospital and in Boston the common threads are easy to find. She provided medical history when they needed it and she asked questions. Intelligent and well thought out questions based on her knowledge of Janet and her medical conditions. Her knowledge of her mother magically produced the right questions at the right time and did not offend the medical folks because she was credible. Credibility did not come from debating, or even discussing, medicine. She was speaking the common language of the patient. The result was that those professionals took the time to provide a higher level of care for Janet. That would not have happened if Jennie did not prepare for her role as Janet's advocate or if she did not treat the medical professionals with the respect they deserved.

Jennie did her homework. Knowing what questions to ask was not hard. What if you have not done the preparation work, you're emotionally overwhelmed or just can't think of what to ask? In my search for a healthcare advocacy handbook, one of the best bits of advice I found came from Dr. Groopman. He suggests that by asking questions "...a patient, friend, or family member can slow down the doctor's pace and help him think more broadly." How many times in a discussion has someone asked you a question and you magically remembered something important to the conversation? (As you get older it will happen a lot more.) He suggests asking questions such as:

1. What else could be causing this?

2. Is it possible that there could be more than one problem?

3. Is there anything that does not fit in?

4. What other body parts are near it?

5. What is the worst thing this can be?

6. I know Dad has some medical conditions. What could this be if it is not one of those? [44]

We have also learned a few that work well:

1. Has mom been tested for that before?

2. Is there anything about the test(s) that is unclear?

3. Are there any other symptoms that we should be looking for?

4. Is there any other information I can give you that might help?

5. I have a summary of Mom's medical history here, would you like a copy?

I am sure you can think of dozens more. The key is that we're not asking about medical esoterica from the internet, we're asking about Mom or Dad. When you're engaged in Mom's care, some of the greatest questions will just come to you in the most basic ways.

## The Person in Charge

One day while walking to the intensive care unit (ICU) waiting room of a local hospital I observed a young woman, I'd say late 20's to early 30's. She was talking with one of the hospital case managers (we've seen case managers called social workers and discharge planners and I am sure there are more titles for the job). The young woman was fighting tears, nodding her head in agreement, but not looking very sure of anything. The case manager was talking in a sincere muted voice while maintaining near constant eye contact. Even if you didn't know the players, in any context, an authority was offering information to someone in need.

When sitting in the ICU waiting room shortly after, the young woman came in and sat with her back to mine. After controlling her tears, she called her mother to update her on the condition of their loved one, her father. I gathered my things and was getting up to move to sit out of earshot, when I could not help but overhear one side of the cell conversation:

He's about the same. *pause* No, he didn't know me. A hospital person came to talk with me. *pause* Not sure. *pause* Not about insurance. She talked about making one of us the power of attorney, advance directives or something like that. She said one of us or both of us can do it. It would make it so we can make decisions for dad. I think she was a lawyer. *pause* Don't know. *pause* Wait a minute. She gave me a card. Says case manager. *pause* I don't know Mom. She's the person in charge. *pause* Not a doctor or nurse. She works in the office. *pause* Mom, I don't know. Maybe she's a lawyer and a case manager. *pause* Talks like a lawyer (*disgusted daughter sigh*). *pause* I don't know Mom. You can talk to her when you get here.

⁓

The young woman and her mother were about to make some major decisions that they were not prepared to make. If a case manager comes to talk to you and you do not understand what their job is or have any clue about the implications of the actions they are suggesting, they do come across like the person in charge and they do sometimes sound like lawyers. They are not in charge and they're not lawyers.

Unless you've done the work to prepare in advance, when the case manager comes to see you, or you go to your first meeting with them, you are at a serious disadvantage. You are at your worst. The case manager already has a plan for how this is all going to play out, what choices that you and your loved one should make (in the case manager's judgment) and the choices the administration and the insurance company want you to make. You are worried about your loved one, scared, beyond stressed, not familiar with the subject matter and likely at the point of vulnerability. You're ready to open up and swallow whatever you're told by a person of apparent authority. Who are these folks so concerned about the advance directive (or DNR) and why do they have the case manager talking to you about it now? You have gone through the process of helping Mom and Dad make informed decisions about care when they are sick and at their deaths and you have the paperwork properly in place, when the case manager comes to you, take a deep breath, tell her what the documents say and remind her that she already has copies of them. Relax, you've got this.

Case managers are almost always nurses who did that for awhile and don't anymore. They're always overworked and stuck shuffling a lot of paper all day, every day. They can be your best friend or the biggest pain in the system. An adversarial case manager can negate all of your effectiveness along with the good work of the medical workers caring for Dad with a heart breaking walk-off home run.

When your loved one is discharged from the hospital, they either go home, to a rehabilitation facility, assisted living arrangement or a nursing home. Either way, there is planning that has to be done to insure that wherever they go their conditions can be cared for, the odds are greatest they will continue to recuperate and that they are safe. If that can't be done, Dad can't leave. He cannot be wheeled to the curb without a plan (or at least what passes for one). The case manager puts the plan together. Their job is to work with other facilities, home care organizations and the family to see that the patient's healthcare needs are met after they leave the hospital.

There is however a factory piece-work element to the case manager job. As always, the business of medicine is applying force to move Mom along in the most cost effective way. Add to that the long list of patients the case manager is trying to get discharged, free up beds for more patients and do so using medically accepted methods all the while dealing with the patients and their families. It's easy to see the importance of a good working relationship with the case management folks. When that's not possible, you have to get creative.

⌒

Janet spent several months in a long-term acute care hospital (LTACH) in the greater Boston area. The LTACH to Janet was effectively a specialized pre-rehab. She was placed there for their respiratory expertise.

It was the case management folks at the Brigham that selected the LTACH based on Janet's complex issues. Among which was that she needed to be weaned from the respirator, learn to walk again and she had to have three dialysis treatments a week. When a case manager looks to place a patient in whatever place is appropriate, they have to make sure that things like respirators and dialysis treatments are accounted for. Sending Janet to the same sports rehab as one of the Boston Celtics just because they like her insurance and have an open bed won't work. She could not do the work and they could not provide the treatments that she needed. She had to go somewhere that she would have a chance to succeed. It just happened that what she needed was rare and about 60 miles from her home.

The folks at the Brigham found a place that could help Janet, transferred all of her records and transported her to the LTACH where she was received, admitted and given a room on the respiratory care floor, a job well done.

Janet made slow but steady progress at the LTACH. She worked hard, there were some setbacks, but she kept getting better in small increments. They don't let you stay in a LTACH (or be an inpatient anywhere other than a nursing home) unless you can show steady improvement and your insurance company will pay for it. Janet had excellent insurance. If the care was medically justified, the insurance company wrote the check. The key for being in a LTACH for so long was the steady improvement she could work toward and achieve. The setbacks were ok, so long as she came back to rehab and started showing that steady improvement again. The problem came when the management of the LTACH decided it was time for Janet to leave.

At the LTACH there were angels, occasionally offset by a person who would stack the raw bedpans in the closet. The staff on the floor was excellent 90% of the time, some of the doctors less than that. It was the administration that presented new challenges for Jennie.

Janet had been at the LTACH for a month or so and was showing steady improvement through reduction of her reliance on the respirator and was able to stand and take a few steps. The New England winter was subsiding and signs of life were popping up at the LTACH.

The physical and occupational therapy folks and the respiratory staff had come to love Janet. Most of the doctors were working with Jennie and seeing value in her presence. The nursing staff found that Jennie was willing to help with minor tasks, freeing them up when the workload was unusually high. If Janet needed something cleaned, was overdue for her bath or needed to go on the bed pan, she'd just do it most of the time. The LTACH admin did not like her efforts, but like any business, a lot goes on that can't be seen from the corner offices.

About 4 weeks in, the case worker, Angelina, started coming around talking about discharging Janet. Jennie and she would discuss Janet's progress and what still needed to be accomplished. Angelina would then say, "well, your mother's insurance will not pay for her to stay here forever" and off she'd go.

Several solo rounds later, she tagged her boss in, Frankie. Angelina was a pleasant middle-aged former nurse/case manager of average height. She typically dressed, acted and even smelled tired. When Jennie would go to her office it was often locked. She was in there, it was just locked. Knocks went unanswered and notes were slid under the door.

Frankie however was going places. She was a walking, talking, middle-aged promotion for a dress for success mini-series. Most women that tall shy away from heels at work. She was a former nurse that confidently engaged in business like only the best on-line MBA graduates can. She knew how to handle Jennie.

Even before her heart surgery, Jennie and Janet were shopping for rehabs. At the time they did not know she'd need an LTACH (or even what one was). They had selected a new rehab about 15 miles from Janet's home. It was a new facility with a lot of big bright windows and a staff that appeared to be perky, pleasant and accommodating. With the addition of the LTACH to Janet's recovery process, the time frame changed but the plan was the same. The day Janet was admitted to the LTACH, Jennie dutifully (if somewhat naively) reported to Angelina that when discharge day arrived, the local facility was ready to take her.

After a few visits from the pair, Frankie and Angelina informed Jennie that in 4 days Janet would be discharged and sent to a rehab in a town about 40 miles from her home. She was told that the local rehab selected by Janet did not have a bed for Janet and this other place did. We later learned that the local rehab had not been called, but when we looked into it she would not have been admitted because of her remaining conditions and her inability to meet the daily requirements for physical therapy.

Jennie and I went to visit the new rehab selected by Frankie. It was a huge facility, quite impressive. We met with a very nice case manager who was handling the intake paperwork and she gave us a tour. It was more like a health resort than a rehab and was closer to home. It was also a much easier drive so Jennie might be able to come home most nights. We were less skeptical and I was getting optimistic. Jennie asked to see the dialysis unit and about their respiratory department. We were told they did not have capabilities for those conditions and that she did not know Janet had them. After our march back to her office, we all could see that the screening package from the LTACH did not mention her respiratory issues or her need for 3 dialysis treatments a week. That put an end to Janet going there, but not Frankie's eviction proceedings.

Knowing that Janet was going to be discharged soon, we started our own pre-screening process. I looked up every rehab within 150 miles of Janet's home. If there was even a chance they could handle the respiratory issues and at least transport her for dialysis I called them. The plan was to visit all possible rehabs before Frankie could ship her off to the first one with an available bed. We quickly learned that there was no rehab (other than a different and more distant LTACH) that could provide the care that Janet needed. After too many hours and much debate, the LTACH case management team also concluded that there was no other place for Janet than in their facility. Frankie and her staff were not happy. Jennie's focus returned to her mother and I stopped interrogating rehabs.

Both of Janet's parents were ministers, Jennie's dad studied for the ministry and Jennie was raised in a strong Christian environment. It was woven into their lives. Jennie found comfort in having her lunch just outside the door to the chapel at the LTACH. She could pray inside before or after eating and it all made for nice quiet time for her. About two weeks after the first discharge fire-drill, Jennie was eating outside the chapel. Frankie and Angelina knew she would be there and marched on over to present her with a bill for $81,200.00. Jennie was told that the bill was for the 14 days since Janet's discharge date and that she was being charged $5,800.00 per day from then on because her insurance would not pay beyond the discharge date.

Remembering that the insurance company's case manager only gets what the provider case manager sends to them, Jennie and I called Janet's insurance case manager. We told her of our plight and were informed that coverage had been stopped because Janet "refused" to go to the facility that Frankie wanted to send her to. After explaining what had occurred, the insurance company agreed to revisit the situation. I requested and received the pages from the insurance company's procedures manual that control a patient's admission and discharge from a LTACH. The five page document revealed that the LTACH had made no attempt at compliance from the moment Janet was admitted. While the one from your loved one's provider may not read exactly like Janet's, what it controls will likely be similar but tailored for the ICUs, hospitals, rehabs and nursing homes. It covers, what conditions are accepted (clinical indications for admission), an overview of the course of recovery, requirements for evaluation and treatment, discharge criteria and discharge planning. Two full pages of the five laid out the rules for discharge planning. It's obvious that there are standards of care that control where your loved one goes, when and why. It did not take a medical degree or an insurance professional to see that, without a plan that included a place to send Janet where her conditions would be cared for, the LTACH couldn't discharge her and the insurance company would keep paying the bill. Based on our research, and that of the case management staff's, there was no less costly place for her to go. They had stopped Janet's coverage based on the same misinformation that caused Frankie's rehab selection to accept her. I guess it all could be one big misunderstanding or coincidental oversights and not the malicious actions of a damaged case management supervisor. We'll never know, but it was far from over.

In a family meeting with more staff than family (it always works out that way when they're not happy with you), we were told that the days that were not covered by the insurance company still had to be paid by Janet ($135K +/- at that point). The LTACH admin folks knew well that once it was shown that Janet was never ready for discharge to Frankie's rehab and that there was no other facility that could accommodate her conditions, that those days would be covered. They just found it more entertaining to make their threat in front of all of Janet's family so that the billing scare would continue, even if that meant that Janet had to needlessly hear and worry about it also.

At the meeting they also informed us that Janet was totally coming off the respirator that day and her conditions had improved to the point that she could now be safely discharged to another facility or maybe even go home. This was not the case, but they were the medical experts and had filed their reports.

Family meetings sometimes include a representative from some or all of the departments that are treating your loved one. The physical and occupational therapy folks agreed that the work they were doing could be done in a conventional rehab, eventually in an outpatient facility or even at home. The respiratory staff was concerned that even if she was off the respirator, the opening for it (the stoma) would still be in her throat and it needed skilled care until it healed up, but they were willing to discharge her if the right services were available where she was going. The head of nephrology, Dr. Fitzgerald felt that, if the only issue was her dialysis treatments, she might be ready to go to a rehab or even home with the right preparations, but all of her conditions combined would make going home unsafe at that point.

Only one doctor addressed all of Janet's conditions. This happens because each specialty area of medicine tends to exist in their own little fiefdoms. Frankie was able to dissect Janet's status into small justifications for her discharge but only Dr. Fitzgerald (who had his own fiefdom to manage) was able to look at the patient as a whole.

The medical director was often in the halls, Jennie saw him on the floor most every day. When asked for a meeting with him, it took almost a week to sit him down. When we did talk, he supported case management's position that it was time to move Janet along. When asked about Dr. Fitzgerald's opinion, we were told that he was alone in thinking that Janet was not ready to be discharged. When asked what the insurance company thought of his opinion, he said that he did not know what had been communicated to them.

Dr. Fitzgerald offered to speak with the insurance company directly. After a few calls with the medical review team at the insurance company, it was decided that because there was no other possible facility that could handle her conditions, that she would stay at the LTACH until she was ready to go home or until she stopped improving. We had no idea what a medical review team was, but we were not going to forget about it. A medical review team, in this situation, was a group of medical professionals working for or associated with the insurance company that looked at the medical facts and offered a 3rd party opinion on the care needed and thus paid for, the court that overruled Frankie.

Being the medical historian, knowing what mom wanted and showing up was not enough. Being nice and trying to tactfully engage with the case management folks trying to discharge Janet failed also. This worked out for Janet because we asked questions. We did not make demands or blow things up, we asked questions. The answers we received clearly saved Janet major discomfort, stress and very likely medical complications from being placed in a facility unable to care for her correctly. Our questioning helped the medical workers do their jobs better.

## Discharge Planning

The importance of a good working relationship with the case manager cannot be overstressed. As soon as your loved one is admitted, the insurance company and the facility are planning for their discharge. If they aren't, policy and procedure states they should be. On Mom's first day in the hospital, find out who the case manager is going to be and go meet her. Get her business card and ask if she is the only person who will be following your mother throughout her inpatient stay. (Please forgive the apparent sexism, I've never met a male case manager.)

This is a process. If your mom is going to a rehab when she is discharged, you do not want to be surprised to learn that she is going to a facility 50 miles away because that is the only bed (or first available) they can find for her. That may be the reality, but you need to be on top of what is happening. The case manager is going to assemble your mom's file and send it to rehabs. That is so they know what conditions and special requirements your mom has. If they aren't equipped or staffed to properly care for her, she can't go there. That is called screening and it can be a very rushed part of the process. Case managers are always busy and if they can find a bed for Mom with one call, why make more? Ideally, you would know which facilities Mom is being screened for and have the time to visit them before hand or at least Google them and call to make sure they are truly prepared for her. The screening process is also a bit of a chess game. It may be impossible to see that Mom gets placed in that great rehabilitation facility that just happens to be near your house, but you can make sure she is admitted to one that can meet her medical needs. If a facility admits a person they are not equipped to handle, it can be a disaster. If someone is recovering from hip surgery also happens to have advanced dementia with the occasional behavioral outburst, it can be an unpleasant awakening for a rehab that is not prepared for that level of care, especially if they can't provide the required additional safety precautions. It is important to have Dad rehab in a place within a reasonable distance from home but it is also important to make sure that he is safe, properly cared for and can succeed there.

Jennie always found it informative to ask the screening rehab to fax or email her the screening packet from the facility trying to send Janet there. You might be amazed at what you read (or not read) in the screening packet. She always made sure the admitting case manager had a copy of her summary of Janet's medical history and current conditions.

If you are involved in the process and know of that really nice rehab across from your favorite coffee shop, you stand a better chance of having her screened there. If you're not in contact with the case manager when they start screening, Mom will be going where the case manager's friend works or someplace whose name begins with the letter A. If your mom has special conditions as Janet did, make sure that wherever she is going knows about them before she is discharged and that facility's level of care is certified to meet her medical needs. If your loved one is discharged to a facility (or home) and their needs for care and safety cannot be met, it would be logical that they would then return to the facility that discharged them. It doesn't work that way. Once discharged, you have to be admitted again and the place you're trying to get Dad back into holds all the cards. All they have to do is say that there is not a bed for him or his conditions do not meet their criteria and you're not getting back in. Do you think that, had Frankie succeeded in discharging Janet when she was not ready, there would be a bed for her when she needed to come back? What would have happened if she had achieved her goal of sending her to the first rehab she could? They would not have been able to handle her conditions and it would have endangered her care and safety. She would have to then be discharged again and admitted to another LTACH. Jennie would have to start all over building relationships with the medical workers in the new facility and Janet would have paid the price.

## Janet Comes Home

Janet was in a tough spot. The medical infrastructure wanted to move her on to less and less costly facilities and eventually home or to a nursing home, but her conditions prevented that for many months. The reality was that she was going to get discharged from the LTACH, it was just a matter of when. Your Mom will not likely have a fraction of the medical requirements that Janet did, but the things we learned from the initial discharge attempts and her eventual return to her home in Maine will provide some insight.

Janet had been weaned from the respirator and was on decreasing

levels of oxygen. It was doubtful as to whether she should ever not
have oxygen bottles around, but the hope was that she would get to
the point that she would not need it all the time. Her mobility had
improved but she was still not able to walk well enough to leave the
LTACH under her own power. She had reached the point where
she was not improving at a rate that could medically justify her existence in the LTACH for much longer. The problem was still finding
a place she could go. Any potential rehab facility would have to have
the ability to handle the dialysis treatments and that proved impossible. We could not even find a nursing home that could handle the
dialysis (not that Janet would have agreed to one or Jennie would
have allowed that to happen). Jennie's plan was to take her home and,
having been away from her home in hospitals and rehab for over a
year, Janet was all for it.

Janet's home was built in 1830 and about as handicap-accessible
as Tarzan's tree house. You could not get a wheelchair through the
doors let alone a gurney. She would need PT and OT to continue at
the house, nurses to come, round the clock care and a way to get to
dialysis. It seemed insurmountable. Jennie was tenacious.

We called Bruce, a friend of the family, man about town, owner of
the best old man truck and the handyman that had worked on Janet's
house for decades. He built an oversized ramp combined with a deck
that Janet could enjoy on warm afternoons with a wide door and
sill that would facilitate all sorts of mobility devices. Being Maine, a
generator was installed to provide electrical backup for the medical
equipment and heating system.

Jennie worked with the insurance company as well. They were always helpful, but when the topic included Janet leaving the $5,800.00

per day LTACH they really stepped up. We learned that the insurance company would support and facilitate medical professionals training family members to do some medical tasks. One such procedure was maintaining the stoma. That was the opening in Janet's throat that was still open from where the respirator tube went in. It would heal over time but it needed to be cleaned more frequently than home nursing services could provide. Due to Janet's severe osteoporosis and multiple transfers in and out of ambulances and to and from hospital beds and hospital tables she developed a breakthrough on the delicate skin of her back which also required specialized wound care. Jennie was trained and certified in the duties of emergency respiratory care, the operation and maintenance of oxygen equipment, wound care and feeding tube hookups and disconnects.

Even Jennie needs to sleep, eat and maintain her sanity. If Janet was coming home, someone needed to be quickly available for her 24x7 for at least the first few months. She did not need ICU level care, but could not be left alone without at least someone in the house with her for long periods of time. There are 168 hours in a week. Jennie was good for 60-80 without burning out completely.

We've seen families in these cases pull together and do amazing things but it's very rare. In most families there's one kid that serves as a caregiver and the rest visit but don't engage as hands-on caregivers. They'll call themselves caregivers, think of themselves as caregivers and often use the "I have to take care of my mother" excuse to get out of other things they justify not doing, but the odds are you're in this alone. If there is nobody else within the family to help, the caregiver child is going to need outside help.

Currently, medical insurance will not pay for caregivers to the extent that Janet needed. Fortunately, she had the foresight to buy and continue to pay into a long-term care insurance policy several years ago. It paid for the extra needed caregivers. Jennie managed a team of caregivers that included a service and private caregivers to fill in the hours that Jennie could not cover effectively. Without her long term care insurance, Janet would have had to spend the family savings to pay for her home care. It is also likely that without it she would have ended up in a nursing home (which is bad enough on its own) and all that her husband and she had worked their lifetime for would have become part of medical industry quarterly profits as opposed to going to their children and grandchildren.

The one remaining issue was the three dialysis treatments a week. There were not a lot of dialysis facilities close to Kittery, Maine, one to be exact. Luckily, it was in the next town over. Janet could not ride in a car yet. On a good day, she could be helped into a wheelchair, but she was still technically bound to a bed or gurney. Wheelchair vans were not covered by her insurance and there were days that she could not be transported in a chair. The only other choice was by ambulance, round trip, three times a week. It would not be covered by her medical or long-term care insurance. If it were covered, the ambulance company would be billing about $3,000.00 for each 14 mile roundtrip. I have no clue what the price would be for Janet to pay out-of-pocket without the benefit of a large insurance industry negotiated rate. She could not afford either rate. It seemed as if we had a deal breaker. I had become accustomed to using Google to find deals on used medical equipment and was soon on Craig's List looking at used ambulances.

As badly as I wanted to drive that Cadillac meat wagon from

Ghostbusters, it was not to be. In one of our conversations about bringing Janet home, we remembered that magic phrase from back at the beginning, when Janet was in the local hospital for her initial heart valve replacement surgery, *medical necessity*. The language of most health insurance allows for some level of apparent deviation from the rules based on a showing of a medical necessity. If a doctor says it is medically needed, sometimes things that the policy appears to prohibit get covered. If the treatment in question is less costly than the alternative, a doctor's written order can be all that is needed, sometimes.

Once again, Janet's nephrologist in Boston, Dr. Fitzgerald, came to Jennie & Janet's rescue and wrote a letter explaining the medical necessity of Janet being transported via ambulance to dialysis at that point in time and the exception was granted. The insurance company would cover the transportation, but there would be regular reviews to make sure it continued to be medically necessary. Dr. Fitzgerald's letter was most influential, but that does not explain the business proposition of it all. It was clear that going home was more cost effective than the LTACH and there was no other place that could handle her conditions within 150 miles of her home. The insurance company could not deny her dialysis treatments. The approval of Janet's transportation costs were never explained to us. It is not hard to deduce why it worked. There was no other place that could provide the care that Janet needed and Jennie was willing to coordinate and participate in all the required home care training/certifications. In light of those facts, and the insurance companies roughly $150,000.00 a month payments to the LTACH, $36,000.00 a month for ambulance rides was clearly a cost effective solution.

All Janet's ducks were in row, the house was prepared, Jennie was trained, extra caregivers were hired and her conditions were planned for. It would seem to most that all that remained was the actual discharge and a ride home.

The discharge plan is really a treatment plan that starts when your loved one leaves a facility. If every time someone at the inpatient facility caring for your loved one even hints at discharge, your mind goes straight to questions about the treatment plan after discharge, you'll do just fine.

Before the time comes to wheel your loved one out, there is a lot of paperwork to be done. The case manager has to make sure that documents are prepared for the medical folks who will be caring for Mom or Dad in the rehab or at home, doctors orders from the discharging facility have to be included, medications have to be accounted for (new prescriptions written and medication lists provided) and instructions for the family have to be reviewed with them and the patient. Regardless of how well this has been planned for, the actual discharge is most likely going to be delegated to a nurse who has far too much to do already. You could end up being handed a stack of papers as they yell "goodbye" when your loved one is being wheeled out by an orderly. You need to slow that process down. Make sure that the case manager and the head nurse on the floor know that you want to sit down and go over the discharge paperwork before Dad is wheelchaired into the hallway holding his plastic bag of belongings. You need to pay special attention to the medication list; get a copy of the discharge summary report and copies of all doctors' orders and written Rx prescriptions; and take the time to sit and study them.

If the discharge plan is not correct, your life will be hell. If all of the things that the discharging facility told you were needed are not in the discharge papers they will not happen. If you're told that Mom needs a visiting nurse to see her three times a week and that is not in the discharge paperwork, the nurse will not be showing up. The discharging facility has no responsibility to correct it after you leave. She is no longer their patient. She's been discharged. Stop NOW and get it fixed and reprinted, you will be glad you did. If you don't, you'll need to contact Mom's PCP, explain the whole mess, they will have to research it and likely want to see her before anyone will write the order for the nurse to come to the house. What if the discharging facility forgets to prescribe oxygen, dialysis treatments or a critical medication? The more involved Mom's conditions are and her treatment is, the more attention you have to pay to the discharge dance.

## Medication Madness

Janet had been moved from the ICU at the local hospital to a room in the step-down unit, a sort of half-way house between ICU and the regular hospital floor. Jennie was in Janet's room when an unfamiliar nurse came in with a small cup filled with pills. That was unusual. Typically, they bring in a tray of medications all sealed in little packages as dispensed by the robotic pharmacist out in the hall and then they open them one at a time. I guess dumping them all in a cup is how they used to do it in the 70s or 80s when the nurse was trained. Janet asked to see them and with a sigh the nurse handed her the cup. Jennie looked and saw that some of them were of colors she had not seen before. When asked why, the nurse responded, "I don't know, those are her meds. Do you want water or juice?" Jennie noted that some did not look right and asked her to find out what they were. She explained that was impossible as she had thrown out the packaging for them. Jennie then insisted that she get another set of packaged pills so that they could verify the ones in the cup. The nurse was not happy, left the room and sent the supervisor in. A battle ensued but, to make a long story short, new pills were brought in and 1/3 of the medications in that first small cup were incorrect. How does that happen? Janet was in the same hospital, she had only moved less than 150 feet from the ICU to the step-down unit. She was on the same floor. The robotic pharmacists are all on the same computer network. She had been "discharged" from the ICU and "admitted" into the step-down unit. That meant that someone had to re-enter into the system her medications list. It was simple preventable human error.

Every time Janet suffered a setback in rehab she would be discharged and admitted to Massachusetts General Hospital or the Brigham and then when she went back to the rehab, she was again discharged and admitted. Not one time in any discharge/admission were the medications ever 100% correct. Medication management is a never ending challenge for the industry. Most medication errors are harmless. They always seem to get the critical ones right, but what if they don't? Stay on top of the medications all the time, at home, inpatient and everywhere in-between.

## *Induced* Confabulation

When my mom was first diagnosed with Alzheimer's, her neurologist explained *confabulation*. It means "to fill in gaps in memory with fabrication."[45] He used the term to show me how Mom could have a conversation with someone she did not remember about a subject she only remembers bits and pieces of and have it make complete sense to anyone listening. Friends and family had no idea that she was subconsciously filling in all the gaps that she had forgotten by making it up as she went along. The problem is that only the person talking with Mom was actually having a conversation. Mom's subconscious mind was spastically trying to help her appear to have a clue about what was being said, she was just trying to get through it. The smile you got when you walked in the room was the only time you really knew Mom remembered.

We have all nodded our head and agreed with someone when we have no idea what they are talking about. Though not to the degree Mom did it, I see many older people doing it, I've heard them saying that they understand or remember but know very well they don't. Little kids do it all the time when they think you're mad at them.

Some medical workers come to rely on what I'll call induced confabulation. They will have no hesitation about talking way to fast and using words that you have no way of understanding. The technique works best from a position of power. They'll often ask you to sit down while they remain standing and then raise their voice slightly. Like Mom, I do not think that they are consciously doing it. They are too busy for your questions and they have been conditioned to instinctively know that when you're intimidated you'll either understand the answer more quickly when they get assertive or that you will be too scared to ask for further clarification. It works very well. The older and more feeble the patient, the better it works.

If you do not understand the explanation that is given to you by a medical worker, keep asking questions until you do. They won't get overly angry (if they do, you're talking to the wrong one). The busy doctor or nurse might let out a disgusted sigh but they will likely also sit down next to you and explain it better. If they don't, ask them when they might have time to talk about Mom. You don't need them to be nice, just communicative.

## *Personality*

When gathering info for this chapter I asked Jennie for a list of the simple things she learned while caring for Janet that anyone can do, regardless of the patient's conditions. Naturally she provided all of the ones listed here, she also wrote: "Be Polite, Respectful but display certainty and resourcefulness."

Reading the words be polite and respectful were not a surprise. It is the instruction to "display certainty and resourcefulness" that made me think. Jennie inherently acts more decisively than I do. Depending on the side of the bed you sleep on, I can be interpreted as being either too reserved or prudently thorough. Regardless, the point is that people have different styles when it comes to interpersonal skills and thus advocacy.

While we need to find a way of working with those that are caring for Mom and Dad, and they may not be all that accustomed to or see a need for working with us, we do have a role to play in our parents care. When you are the medical historian, have helped your parents make informed decisions about their end of life choices, and are actively participating in their care, you are entitled to display certainty in what you know about Mom and Dad. You also have the tools to be just as resourceful as you've come to know Jennie to be. It is a balance you have to find, but if you can find a way to be two parts Jennie and one part Mike, you'll do just fine.

## Short 'n' Sweet

The following are a few items from Jennie's tool bag:

**1. When Mom or Dad is an inpatient at a medical facility, keep on top of those medications and appointments. They won't always tell you what's going on. They're used to families not caring enough to engage, especially in a rehab or nursing home. Get a copy of the medications list each week and compare it to the last. You'll often find that Dr. X came to see Dad and changed everything. I've seen doctors in rehabs and nursing homes just take out all non-essential (in their minds) medications under the heading of decreasing a patient's fall risk.**

When you put a dementia patient in a rehab after surgery to repair a broken hip and take away their medications without finding another one and transitioning them, nothing good is going to come from that. Withdrawing from medication(s) is only going to make an already anxiety ridden and thoroughly uncomfortable experience worse. Arguably, being more emotionally unstable would make for an even greater fall risk. I wonder if simply removing all the meds is really the best thing for the patient or the result of liability management consultants?

If your loved one is in a rehab following surgery, the surgeon and maybe others are going to want to see them, probably before they are discharged from the rehab. The folks at the rehab are not used to you. They operate on the assumption that you view your loved one's time in rehab as a sort of purgatory for them and a time of minimal effort on the family's part. The surgery was not a failure and now they have to recuperate. To most families, this is the time to visit one day on the weekend and call when they think of it. The rehab folks are far more used to hands-off adult children than they are effective advocates. The rehab folks will schedule appointments, load Mom in a van, take her to them, load her back in the van and bring her back to the room and you'll never know about it. You need to make it clear to everyone that you need to be at those appointments. They are only slightly less important than the ones where she was diagnosed or consulted on in the ER.

**2. If you're loved one is coming home from a rehab or hospital, there are likely preparations to be made to insure their safety. Perhaps they can live alone or maybe they'll need medical and caregiver support to some degree and the odds are you're going to be a part of whatever team is needed. Make sure you have copies of the discharge papers and doctor's written orders for home nursing, occupational and physical therapy and home health aides.**

There is a trick to managing the home services. They're trying to pack as many home visits into a day as the insurance companies will pay for. The home health aid, nurse, physical therapy and occupational therapy folks are all trying to fill their day in such a way that they meet their job requirements and get home early. They can very well end up coming in one immediately after the other, like a fire drill, to Mom's house every 45 minutes for the entire morning. We've seen them sitting in their cars lined up in the driveway impatiently waiting their turn to get in and out as quickly as possible. When that happens, the treatments will not be effective and Mom will be exhausted before lunch. You know what she can and cannot handle. Slow them down. Tell them she's 85 and can't do 4 appointments in 3 hours. If they have a problem, just say no. Move them to the next day. If Mom is better in the mornings or afternoons, schedule accordingly. You may not always get what is best for Mom, but more often than not you will.

**3. You have preparations to make too. Does Dad have new accessibility needs?**

Do you have to:

A. **Pull up rugs and remove other tripping hazards;**

B. **Clear out space in rooms for a walker or wheelchair so that he can more easily move around;**

C. **Have a wheelchair ramp built, a handicap-accessible tub/shower or stair lift installed;**

D. **Arrange for the proper medical devices and durable medical equipment (DME) like oxygen, a commode, raised toilet seat, bed and chair alarms, video monitors, wheelchair, transport chair (the one with the small wheels, great for use whenever you're not lifting a wheelchair up over stairs) and walker(s);**

E. **Is his bed and other furniture still going to be appropriate (safe for him to use);**

F.  **If home health aides are going to be bathing him, do you have one of those shower heads with a hose;**

G.  **Install grab rails/bars for assistance throughout the residence, and,**

H.  **If caregivers are going to be needed, have you arranged for either a service or private caregivers?**

These are just some of things you might find yourself needing. You are going to be very busy and stressed during and just after the discharge. It is far easier to plan for and deal with these needs before you get home. If you don't, it will be overwhelming. To know what you need, talk with those caring for Mom. The physical and occupational therapy folks know this stuff, start asking them long before the case manager starts talking about discharge.

Medical insurance may cover some of these things. The Lions Clubs in some towns have DME equipment programs where you can go and sign out what you need and then just bring it back when you're done (they are also a great place to donate DME equipment when you don't need it). Amazon is a great place to get as good a price as you're going to find on DME gear, but make sure it's what you want. Many DME items and supplies cannot be returned, even when they are still sealed in the original packaging. I am sure there is at least one DME provider in your area. It is a very profitable segment of the medical industry and most of the items require no medical certifications or training to sell. The local dealer might be the most expensive way to go, but you get what you pay for. They will have a showroom, take some returns, know the product, can advise you on what to get, deliver, install and service it when it breaks. If you didn't know what DME was until the last couple pages, go see your local dealer. Your life will be much easier.

**4. The business of medicine will make sure that Mom is not in the hospital any longer than need be.**

It does not always work that way in a rehabilitation facility. You need to keep track of why she is still in the rehab. A close friend of ours that had advanced dementia was in a rehab recovering from hip surgery (he fell down while getting out of bed). We were helping the family deal with medical folks and Jennie was in her defacto health-care advocate mode. After three weeks in the rehab, it seemed like his mobility was as good as it was before his fall and it was expected he'd be discharged soon. The staff had said on several occasions that there was not much else they could help him with and his dementia combined with the staffing ratios made it safer for him to be at home. Knowing which day they like to discharge patients and having made all the needed preparations in his home for his family to care for him, Jennie asked about the impending discharge. She was told that they were keeping him another week. When asked what they hoped to accomplish, she was told "nothing, the insurance will pay for it so we're keeping him." I still laugh when I think of it. Yes, they had empty beds, it is a business, they could have justified writing reports and orders so that the insurance company would pay for it, but damn, is billing another week really worth the risk to the patient? There is also the possibility that the rehab folks are just so used to us wanting to keep our parents in purgatory that they are conditioned to keep them as long as the insurance will pay for it.

**5. My Dad and every other senior that I've cared for gets con-fused and anxious some of the time. When you're not going to be there it helps to type and print them a note. In a large clear font tell them:**

A. What is going on, what you'll be doing and where you will be when they read the note for the 10th time while you're not there (even if you just told them 3 times before you left);

B. Tell them what's going to happen next, who's going to be coming to see them, when they're coming and when you'll be back;

C. Include the next scheduled appointment they have, if you're taking them or who will be, what time the appointment is and when they'll be picked up;

D. Don't forget to detail any other things you'll be doing before or after the appointment (lunch, breakfast or some errands);

E. Tell them that you love them, put your phone number(s) on it in a large font, maybe put one copy near where they sit in living room, kitchen and next to their bed; and,

F. Don't forget to remove the old notes when you give them new ones. When you do give them the new one, they will want to read it and confirm with you at least once what the note says—be patient.

Following that same logic, print large font calendars with upcoming appointments, birthdays, important events and the like. Yes, it's just a calendar, but it's a calendar that you prepared and keep updated for them. It makes yet another important connection for them. It makes them feel safer.

**6. Keep several copies of your short list of their conditions and medications around. Hand them out to medical workers during admission, to everyone on the floor treating them and post one on the wall along with your signs.**

If you asked my mother if she drove, did her own shopping, cooked her own meals, had good balance and was totally independent, she would tell you in a most convincing way that she did those things and lives alone. If the person knew her and was accustomed to Alzheimer's patients it would not be a problem, but what if it was someone sent to just gather factual information regarding Mom's care? It could have been a problem if they treated or admitted her without a true understanding of her condition.

You know fact from fiction, others might not. In your summary of Mom's recent medical history and current medications include any fiction the medical providers are likely to hear from your loved one.

When Jennie was helping our dementia suffering friend after his hip surgery, she handed out one of those summaries to every medical worker caring for him and many commented on how they wished everyone would do that. When she met with the case manager at the rehab prior to his admission, she offered one to her and was told that she already had a copy, that it was a great idea and wondered where it came from. The discharging case manager at the hospital had included it in the screening package.

Along the same lines, when going to appointments with your loved one, bring at least two copies of your medical history summary. Offer one to the doctor, "this is a copy of my notes on my mother, would you like to see it?" Nobody does that. They won't be able to resist looking at it. If you've done your preparation well, they'll comment on it and ask to keep it. It's not a medical record, but it is what they need. It's more efficient.

**7. Regardless of Mom and Dad's age or conditions, nothing happens in a vacuum. Even the simplest stay in a medical facility is much more difficult than it would be for you. They become confused. Mom's not in her home walking around on her floors wearing her slippers. She's alone in a hospital bed, with a roommate, and walking on highly polished floors with socks that have grippers on one side, but when they are on inside out, they're roller-skates.**

This is an uncertain time for anyone and a scary one for Mom or Dad. Things like anesthesia and medication changes can have a much more severe effect on an older person. Even seniors that are still sharp as a tack can suffer some temporary loss of cognition after being under anesthesia. There is not much you can do to compensate for these issues other than to be the aware and consistent healthcare advocate that Mom needs.

**8. You'll be much less frustrated if you don't hold others to your standards, especially family and friends. You've made a decision to do this for your parents and are doing the best you can. You'll only get even more stressed with the process if you continually expect help from family and friends that won't. If they pitch in**

and help, that's awesome. It will be far better for Mom, Dad and everyone involved if the family shares in the experience, but that is very unlikely. The odds are it's going to be you alone, doing it all. You're not going to change your family, why stress and fume over what you can't control?

**9.** Many health providers now have patient portals that often provide access to a patient's recent medical records, such as visit notes and test results. Set up access and use the portals.

**10.** Patients are often not told how to take medications, about side effects or sometimes even when to take them and how many to take.[46] When a doctor prescribes something new, ask them for details about the new drug and if you should be looking for any side effects or interactions with Dad's other medications. They have software and phone apps that check for those things, but do not assume the doctor and any of their busy staff took the time to use them or read the results. When you pick up the new prescription at the pharmacy, don't just grab it and head for the frozen pizza and wine aisles. Ask the pharmacist the same questions.

**11.** The time will come when it is not safe for Mom and Dad to drive any longer. This can be a huge issue. For our parents, the automobile is freedom, one of their last bastions of independence. When we're old, we'll just grab our phones and text Geri-Uber. Mom and Dad's minds don't work that way. Driving your own car is sacred. When the time comes that you think safety is an issue, don't be the heavy. Let his or her PCP be the bad guy. You have to put in place the proper documents that en-

**able you to communicate directly with the providers. Call the PCP and tell them of your concerns and ask them to evaluate Mom or Dad to see if it is safe for them to drive. If it's not, they know how to handle it. It won't be pretty and the cops may get involved, but that only makes for better stories later on. Dad will be furious with his PCP for a while, maybe a long time, but you won't have been the one to deprive him of his freedom.**

## Breathe

As your parents' advocate, the decisions that you make will be either emergent, needing immediate response, or you'll have time to think about it, check your notes and even do some research. Other than deciding to dial 911, I doubt you'll ever have to make an emergent decision. In those situations, the medical folks, be they the staff at an inpatient facility or EMTs, will not be looking for your input. Other than directing them to the File of Life and stating that Dad does or doesn't have a DNR, there is not much you can do.

Aside from the rare emergency, you will have time to think. You never have to make snap decisions. When getting barraged by medical folks as well as friends and family it is only natural to get overwhelmed by emotion. If you don't know what a panic attack feels like, you might find out. Take your time. Breathe deep. Having prepared properly, you have all of your loved one's healthcare choices documented and you know well what they want. You are their advocate. Stop, think, use your resources, you know what to do.

## Chapter Eight

......................................

# The Dying

While there is a lack of detailed information out there to guide you in your healthcare advocacy efforts for Mom and Dad, there is no shortage of information on death. The problem with the plethora of solid information on dying is that even if we do read it, we don't seem to get it. We can choose to ignore or deny death, but it's not going anywhere. We have refined the art of gallows humor to facilitate not dealing with it. Even when we try to be serious, death isn't spoken of directly, just alluded to, "Mom's not getting any younger" or "Dad won't be around forever" and so on.

When we spend money on Wills, Trusts, financial planning and other things that come under the common heading of estate planning we tell ourselves that we are preparing for death. That may be somewhat true, but we are also denying it. Arranging our affairs is a wise and healthy thing to do, but we're also allowing our death terrors a fieldtrip to enjoy a subconscious attempt to control what we cannot.

If that were not true, as consumers, we would not settle for what we're sold. We'd expect our attorneys and the medical industry to engage in the end of life healthcare decision making beyond cutting and pasting something together and throwing it in with the deluxe package or, in the case of healthcare providers, using the form in the drawer that's barely legible because it's been copied a hundred times or more.

My experience has been that your parents are more comfortable talking about dying than you are. I doubt they're looking forward to it, but from what I have seen, most seniors are able to talk about it. When we introduce the idea of informed end of life choices to clients, it's the under 60 crowd that gets evasive about the process. Some just refuse to listen, stating that the simple form with the check boxes is all they need. Others initially state that they don't want to deal with it, they then take the paperwork home and later decide that it's not such a bad idea after all. My parents were fine talking about dying and I have not worked with an older person who had a problem planning for it. The kids however, that's a different story. The tissues on the table in my office are not there for the parents. When we ask older folks what their children think about they're getting older and dying, it is not uncommon to hear "my daughter (or son) just cries whenever we bring it up" or the more tactful "they're not ready to talk about it yet."

You need to deal with why you are so uncomfortable talking about Mom and Dad dying. If you do, you'll make the whole process easier for them (not to mention yourself). If you can get over yourself enough to talk openly with them about death, everything leading up to the day they die will be a far better experience for all of you and the grieving will be far less painful. It works that way when you are engaged in the process with them and not just on the sidelines denying reality and waiting to be kicked in the head.

If you can't talk to Mom and Dad about death, your advocacy efforts will not be nearly as successful and you'll miss out on the experience of helping them when they need you the most. If you don't engage in the process, all of it, you won't get to have that wonderfully peaceful ah-ha moment when you stop crying and say to yourself, "that weird guy, the one with the book about helping our parents, he was right, it was a rewarding experience that I would never have been able to share with my parents if I had not engaged in their medical care and deaths. It doesn't hurt nearly as bad as I expected and I'm handling it far better than the rest of the family."

There is a strategic reason to engage in Mom's care as she approaches death as well. It's not just you that sees Mom is old. In his discussion of the *Exploitation of Death*, Dr. Jay Katz, as a psychoanalyst, remarks that death is the most taboo subject, more so than sex or violence. He also comments that "death has a special place in the practice of medicine...the presence of death is an invisible third party in doctor's offices" and that a doctors silence about death creates discomfort and reinforces his or her authority. Your presence with Mom at appointments, as an active participant in her care, helping her define and affect her choices for care at the end of her life not only negates death as a third party influence but also turns the tables in her favor. [47]

Most families have at least one, that thing that happened years ago. Nobody speaks of it, but it's always there and things are never really as copacetic as they would've been had the issue never arisen or had it been resolved. When someone directly involved dies we say things like "he does not care about that anymore", "she's in a better place now, it does not matter" or "we got over that years ago" but it's still there. In the worst cases, it eats at people and they never fully grieve.

Dr. Ira Byock is a former president of the American Academy of Hospice and Palliative Medicine as well as being the author of *Dying Well*. In the book he wrote about the death of a cancer patient, Ann Marie. Dr. Byock details how Ann Marie's choices for care focused on her quality of life as opposed to trying to buck the tide and have every possible treatment and procedure. She chose to live the rest of her life accepting her fate, "I don't want to spend my last days puking up my guts."[48]

Ann Marie had been very close to her sister when they were young but a man came between them. Once she learned of her sister's fate, Kathy convinced Ann Marie to move in so that she could serve as her caregiver. The process renewed their closeness. As Ann Marie weakened, they became secure in the man of their past's insignificance. How do you think Ann Marie would have felt if she spent her last days or even hours filled with frustration or anxiety, knowing she failed to make things right with her sister? The insignificant man might have never allowed Kathy to let Ann Marie go. By stepping up and caring for her sister, she was able to resolve it for both of them while facilitating their reconnecting at a time when they both needed it the most. Her efforts combined with Ann Marie's logical informed choices about care in her last year made the experience the best that it could possibly have been, for both of them.

The story of Ann Marie does more than illustrate the need to resolve conflicts with those we love while we still can. Her choice to accept the reality of her cancer as opposed to trying every possible treatment and fighting until the very end opens the door for a discussion of medicine's role in such decisions. Dr. Sherwin Nuland cautions us against fighting our fate and blames, in part, the temptation to do so on the nature of those treating us. Doctors are trained to fix things and they are extremely competitive. He explains that the most important ingredient in a doctor's self image is solving the *Riddle*, which is his term for making a correct diagnosis and carrying out a specific cure. He went into medicine after being influenced by a primary care provider that made house calls to visit his dying mother when he was a child. He wanted to be that person who helped his mother, the man that everyone respected and looked up to. When he became a part of the medical industry, the *Riddle* became more important than making house calls and being respected by laypeople. The game was on.[49]

It is a doctor's obsession with the game (solving the *Riddle*) that sometimes enables us to justify any and all treatments as we scramble to cheat death. I get it. If there is any chance to live, hell yeah, real men battle to the end, let's beat this thing, but at what cost? Patients, families and doctors all appropriate the terms living, surviving, quality of life and quality of death very differently and often inconsistently. Without a clear understanding of how everyone involved defines quality of life, I don't see how the patient's best interest can ever be served. Taking the time to define and plan for enjoying a quality of life that we are willing to accept will clearly establish that definition for everyone.

When doctors are in the game and see even the slightest chance to solve the *Riddle*, they are going to tell you that treatment X combined with procedures Y and Z might help you live longer. They might insinuate or mention in passing the possibility or probability that your extended time is going to be spent in misery, but you don't want to hear that. If they succeed in getting a late check out for you, you may well spend your extra hours in a living hell wishing you had never listened to them. They did their job and you let them.

One problem with the never give up attitude is that you get so caught up in it that you forget to say goodbye. The desperate fight for life gets in the way and we forget to die well. By not accepting the inevitability of our death we miss out on the loving closeness shared by Ann Marie and Kathy.

As Mom's effective advocate, you've helped her make informed choices. You know the quality of life she is willing to accept. The two of you have talked about her conditions and how they will affect her death. The process that the two of you engaged in counteracts the medical industry's games and need to solve *Riddles*. It allows Mom to decide how her death is going to play out.

Many commentators have written of the importance of caring for our loved ones when they are sick and at the time of death and all of them note that doing so greatly improves the experience for everyone involved. The closeness that Jennie and I experienced with our parents when caring for them was far from unique. If it is the most loving and least painful way for us to deal with the inevitable demise of our loved ones, why don't we all do it?

Early on in Dr. Byock's medical career he was faced with his father's illness and death. He was able to put aside his medical training and engage with his dad's care just as you will. By being a loving son and caregiver, Dr. Byock was able to look past his training and the medical industry and he wrote of the experience that in addition to being one of great sadness that "Something about that time was also, undeniably precious." He also commented that while caring for his dad that "...as a family we had never been more intimate, more open, or more openly loving" and that the illness forced them to talk about the things that mattered.

He explains that in a teaching hospital (and I suspect most others as well) that "death is always treated as a problem." The doctors have to deal with a Death Summary, inches of forms, a presentation to the Morbidity and Mortality review board and the painful, awkward discussion with the family. Helping his father die provided him with a more loving perspective.[50]

We have this romantic image of holding Mom's hand and telling her how much we love her as she falls peacefully into the forever sleep. The odds are great that it's not going down that way. If you are engaged with her care at the end of her life and you are not there holding her hand the moment she dies, it won't matter. You'll both truly know that you have loved and are going to miss each other. You'll have fully enjoyed your time together and you won't be any more remorseful if Mom dies in her sleep or while you're out walking the dog.

The night Mom died, my brother called. He wanted to bring a friend over to say a prayer that was especially meaningful and asked if she was still up. I had just carried her to bed, but she was more than willing to stay awake for a visit. He arrived with his wife and kids. That crew is hard to corral. Mom was thrilled to have all of them sitting on and surrounding her bed. I went up stairs while they held hands and recited the serenity prayer. When the prayer was over, Mom died.

Mom had completely stopped eating a few days before but was hanging on. She needed to see my brother and his family, all together, in that context, one more time.

I heard my father die through a wireless baby monitor at 4:00 in the morning. Mom and I cared for Dad in their home. He enjoyed visits from the rest of the family that came almost daily. As it became clear that his life would be ending soon, the rest of the family pushed to engage hospice. Further treatment made no sense, he was just worn out. We did agree to home hospice care from a medical standpoint, but we were dragging our heels on the home care services that come with the package.

Dad was eating small amounts of food once or twice a day, coffee in the morning and water when prompted. He was thin and frail. I was not, so I bathed him. He didn't shower. That meant gently lifting him from the wheelchair onto the bath lift, lowering him into the tub, washing the parts he couldn't, then reversing the procedure back into the chair and getting him dressed. Then Jennie would take over.

Every morning, even his last one, I'd get him up with "how ya' doin' Dad?" He'd respond "well, I'm still here Son." That would be followed by a wheelchair ride to the living room and coffee, very hot coffee. Within a few sips, he'd rub his face and ask if Jennie might be around to shave him. Men shave after coffee in the morning. He loved his nice quiet shave in the steamed up bathroom with Jennie. She'd make sure that it was a warm and tender experience. Knowing my father well, Jennie made sure conversation was minimal. He'd get mad when Mom would come home, throw open the door, allowing the warm air out and then irreverently going on about nothing.

Having someone else wash your back is a pleasure. Needing someone to wash other parts of your body shreds your dignity. It took time for Dad to accept Jennie and I caring for him at that level (he did adjust much more quickly to her shaving him than me washing his pits). We were family, it was a loving process filled with humor and radiator-warmed flannel PJs when it was over.

Regardless of the level of care that would have been provided by the workers from the local hospice provider assigned to him, he was about to lose a big chunk of his pride. We were told that I would not be bathing Dad anymore because I was not trained properly, his safety came first. What wasn't disclosed was that giving Dad a shower or sponge bath (no real bath) is a billable expense. In reality, nobody other than me was ever going to bathe him, but Dad heard they were, along with the other services they were going to provide. That meant strangers. I bathed him the night before he died and put him into bed. He slept with two electric blankets, one under the mattress pad and the other on top of the sheet, like a grilled cheese sandwich. The hospice home service lady was coming at 10 the next morning for his scheduled "first bath" but, through sheer will or just good luck, he died before she got there, toasty warm in his own bed.

Some family members and friends have probingly commented on how sad it was that after caring for them as I had that Dad died alone and Mom without me there. I smile. I was more than there, I helped them die. The fact that I was not in the room for Mom's last breath didn't matter. Dad did die when nobody else was in the room, but he did not die alone.

~

I was able to write about my parent's death with ease in about an hour and felt good when I was finished. Janet's took me about a month to get myself mentally prepared for and then another week to get up the strength to hit the keys. I had been telling Jennie for a few weeks that we needed to sit down and go over her memories of the time surrounding Janet's death. I wasn't getting any input, which is unusual. She is always eager to talk about the book, provide details and opinions, proofread things (over and over), and kick me in the butt to complete it. One rainy Sunday morning while handing her the days first cup of coffee, I told her that I was going to write the story of Janet's last few days and asked if we could sit down and talk, to which I got, "I'll have to think about it". Once I sat down to it, the words came quickly and so did the tears. I don't think I cried as much when she actually died. While trying to clear my vision enough to continue typing, an email from Jennie came in. She had been in the other room, writing out her memories, also crying her eyes out. She was right. Neither of us would have been able to sit through a discussion of what happened. It's not the fact that Janet is dead that is so emotional. We talk about her all the time, the good times, the things she did and would be doing as well as her unique behaviors and traits we love and miss. The events of her illness and the challenges that she faced are discussed regularly and even taught as examples in our classes, but we repress the events of her last days. We can easily talk with others about specific details, but putting it all together in our minds and reliving it is sometimes just too much.

## Showdown at the ICU Corral

Janet was in the ICU of the local hospital. The previous week she had been forced against her wishes into DNR status, summoned the strength to reverse it and was then pressured to change her advance directive to one that replaced her well documented end of life choices with those decided by a vote.

Janet's blood pressure would occasionally drop during dialysis. To prevent this they would give her medication before. It dropped one day in the local ICU. Janet and Jennie were out voted on giving Janet the medication to help increase her blood pressure, so dialysis was stopped. It is unsure as to whether Janet was actually given the medication before the treatment. There was also some question as to whether the blood pressure drop was the result of the dialysis or a new blood issue. The kidney doctor (nephrologist), Dr. Sprokette, visited Janet's room. She stated that she would not prescribe the medication or any further dialysis treatments and that "it was time." Janet then looked at Jennie and communicated "time for what?" Dr. Sprokette did not explain anything or attempt to communicate with her in any way other than slapping her with a backhanded death sentence. In Jennie's words "she just talked down to Mom." Janet still had her bean (she knew very well what was going on). There was no question that she had the capacity to make her own decisions but that would not to be allowed any longer.

Jennie excused herself from her mother, chased Dr. Sprokette down the hall and barked at her, "totally unacceptable. You need to respect my mother. She is alert and understands you." Jennie then went on to say that "she has the capacity and the right to make her own treatment decisions. She wants to continue dialysis." This was met with a look of bewilderment and a prompt exit. She never again came to see Janet.

The other agents, under the influence of the majority of the medical staff, had decided enough was enough and it was time to stop dialysis and pull Janet off the respirator. Jennie wanted a family meeting with all of the specialists treating Janet to hear from each of them and then go to her mother and let her decide what was to be done. The family's response was that Jennie was being "ridiculous" and "why do we need a meeting or talk to Mom?" "She signed the papers letting us make the decisions." The medical staff did not explain that Janet retained her mental capacity and under state law still had the right to make her own care decisions until she was deemed to lack that capacity. Everyone was content to blatantly ignore Janet's capacity and allow the family to vote Jennie (and Janet) down whenever doing so fit the business model or satisfied the opinions of others.

The local hospital inconsistently interpreted and adhered to state law as it saw fit, totally independent of any form of oversight. It was all happening far too smoothly. It may not be written in the employee handbook or the policy and procedures manual but this technique was not new to them, it's just the way things are done.

We knew that the only medical person that might possibly still support Janet's choices was the blood doctor (hematologist), Dr. Phillip. There was only one question left, was the blood pressure drop due to the dialysis? If it was dialysis related, it could be treated as it had been for months. If it was a new blood issue, nothing else could be done and, in accordance with Janet's wishes regarding the end of her life, the next step would be to bring her home to die. This was not about whether a medication was properly given or if there was some new undiagnosed blood condition. The real issue was that the medical team had deemed Janet to be a medically futile patient and a waste of hospital resources, again.

The family meeting was agreed to, at which Dr. Phillip would offer his opinion and decisions would be made. We knew that Jennie's efforts to advocate for Janet's wishes had come to an end. Jennie was tortured by the fact that the end of her mother's life would be decided by a vote. She expressed that she was not sure she could be a part of it. I suggested that she not. Jennie had done an amazing job of advocating for her mother's choices for care. Regardless of how informed those choices may or may not have been, Janet had a right to have them adhered to. I suggested to Jennie that we attend the family meeting and if it really was reduced to a vote that she should decline to act as a co-agent under Janet's latest advance directive. I reinforced that she had done all that she could and that I would not want any part of pulling the plug on my mother under these circumstances. She agreed.

We knew well how to prepare for and what to expect from a family meeting. Verbal attacks mixed with emotional dumping by some and medical reports would be presented by others. The last few had been mediated by a palliative care doctor and she had been doing as good a job as possible under the big top. The meetings are usually held in the patient's room or a private office or conference room. There was a meeting room near the ICU where the others had been and we set up in there.

Ten minutes after the appointed time, we sat alone in the room. A few minutes later we were told the meeting was going to be held in the ICU. Jennie stated that her mother should not have to hear this. She was told, "it's not in her room, it's in the ICU." This was different.

As you walk through the security doors into the ICU the patient rooms make up the wall on your left and the counter/desk area is on the right. The pattern flows around the room with space for the medical folks in the middle and the patient rooms in circular fashion around the outside. The doors to the individual ICU rooms have curtains and sliding doors. The idea is that the ICU staff can at least see each patient all the time from the desks in the middle. For the meeting, curtains and sliders were closed on every patient room even close to earshot. To our left and behind us, along the closed patient room sliders, stood the medical staff directly involved with Janet's care. We stood facing into the open space with the security door about 10 feet from our backs. There were a dozen or so people gathered about 15 feet into the room facing us. That group was comprised of staff members not directly involved with Janet's care. We did not know their names but had seen the faces coming and going. They were there for the spectacle, the gallery. Behind us, to our right, stood Dr. Khane and the non-medical folks. The palliative care doctor did not mediate, the medical director and other admin folks were not there. The chaplain with the law degree was.

Everyone knew who we were and why were there, no need for introductions. One by one the specialists walked to the center of the room, standing facing us with the gallery to their backs, each attested to Janet's medical futility.

Then we had to stand in the middle of it all and wait. Dr. Phillip was not there yet. I'd look directly at the folks in the gallery and the medical staff to my left, trying to make eye contact. They were busy inspecting the tops of their shoes. It was clear that Clint Eastwood was not going to show up. The only question was from which door the lions would emerge. This was a show of force, to make it clear that this was their turf, we were not welcome any more and our efforts to advocate for Janet's healthcare choices were over.

It seemed like forever, but it was probably only a couple of minutes before Dr. Phillip arrived. Jennie and I were in a trance, numb, scared and on the verge of tears. It was surreal. Jennie could not speak. I presented the question and Dr. Phillip stated, that nothing more could be done for Janet. I asked whether the blood pressure drop was due to dialysis or blood related. He looked at me for a couple seconds, shook his head, turned his glance to the floor briefly and then left the ICU. I've never felt such silence. Then, from behind, I heard the snide sarcastic "oh, Dr. Jennie, what are you gonna' do now?" followed by giggles and other condescension. When I turned I saw smiling contentment on the face of the heckler and clear support from Dr. Khane, close by, shoulder to shoulder.

The gallery disbursed and a few of the medical folks as well. I told the palliative care doctor that Jennie did not want to participate in the vote and wanted to relinquish her power as agent under Janet's advance directive. Jennie needed to leave. We headed to the chapel. I never really understood the idea of sanctuary until witnessing the value of a hospital's chapel to Jennie. Once they had gathered the papers for Jennie to sign relinquishing her agency power, they knew where to find us.

After the signing we asked about bringing Janet home to die and were told that once the respirator was removed there would not be time to get her there. Our questions as to how they could be certain and why we could not take her home on some combination of oxygen and a portable device went unanswered. The reality was that the others, the medical staff puppet masters and those with preferred voting rights, did not want Janet to die at home. I asked how it would happened, "do they unplug things and give her morphine?" and was told, "no, we don't do that here."

⸺

Nobody else could have done it. Jennie had effectively advocated for her mother for close to two years, she had to be the one to tell Janet. She explained to her that the local hospital would no longer treat her conditions, she could not be transported to Boston this time, and that she would not be allowed to go home to die. Jennie looked at her and asked if she understood, she nodded as a single tear flowed down her left cheek. Jennie explained that she could not be a part of the vote or what was to follow and had signed away her agency power. Through her tears, Jennie said "I love you more than anything. I'm so sorry. I can't help you anymore. After all we've been through." Janet understood and accepted Jennie's words fearlessly but with an exasperated look of total defeat. We said our goodbyes. Between sobs and kissing Janet's hand, Jennie whispered, "I'll see you soon Mom."

⸺

They disconnected life support that afternoon. Janet lived for another 23 hours. I was later told that they gave her morphine to make her comfortable and she died. When I asked previously if they were going to unplug things and give her morphine, I guess I didn't phrase it properly. I forgot the "comfortable" part.

⸺

A couple years later, Jennie ran into Dr. McBride, the heart surgeon that performed Janet's valve replacement who had been so supportive of Jennie as her advocate. He knew well all that had gone on for those two years and asked very matter-of-factly, "was it worth it?" Jennie paused, "It was what Mom wanted. I'd do it again."

Did Janet have a good death? I can see where that could be up for debate. In the sense that she had family around her when she died and a loving and effective advocate throughout her last years, she did have as good a death as was possible considering the circumstances and her choices for care when she was sick and at the end of her life.

Though Janet was not allowed to die in her home as she wished and pretty much lost total control over the last days of her life, she still had Jennie. If she hadn't, none of her choices would ever have been honored and her death would have been facilitated more than two years before when the local hospital decided that doing anything more for her would be futile and a waste of resources the first time. Instead she lived her last two years in medical facilities and at home, constantly hooked up to machines. She never again drove her car, shopped, traveled or put on a food clinic at a breakfast buffet. (I like breakfast, but if you put that woman in a good mid-morning buffet, she'd eat her body weight, rest and go back for more.) The odds are that you may not make the end of life choices that Janet did. You probably couldn't accept the quality of life that Janet had for the last couple years of her life. It's easy for us to say that today.

Before Janet was sick, she lived alone. Her husband had passed and their children were spinning around in the eccentric circles of their own lives. Janet's greatest pleasures were the kids and grandkids.

As with most parents, the lives of her children did not include Janet as much as she would have liked. When Jennie became her advocate, she was around all the time. They became closer. Being sick tends to bring the family together more often and Jennie's siblings also were spending more time with Janet. There was pain and suffering, but she was with her family more and being with her kids and grandkids was the basis for her choice to never give up. Janet was not making choices to get or maintain attention. Her choices were made long before she was sick. The added closeness was a bonus.

I'm pretty sure I could have convinced Janet to change her choices for care. On several occasions I told Janet that I would never go through what she had. In those conversations, she never cut me off or tuned out, she listened attentively. She was tired. I fought the urge to make any attempt to sway her even though I thought that, in the context of any quality of life that I would accept, she should give up. I was tired of being thrown into the family conflicts and seeing my wife verbally bludgeoned by medical professionals, family and friends. I wanted it to end, but more than that, I wanted Janet's right to make choices about her care honored. This is not about our feelings regarding the choices she made, it's about each of us having and keeping control of our lives and deaths.

Janet suffered no loss of cognition. She made choices and properly documented them. Everyone knew what they were. Others decided that, as Dr. Sprokette stated, "it was time." Had she lacked the ability to make her own decisions, this would have been easier to accept. When a patient is in a persistent vegetative state the decision to pull the plug is very different than if they are not. Janet was still watching the 11PM news every night.

At the signing of the last healthcare advance directive, the one that put the end of Janet's life to a vote, the local hospital skipped over the questions regarding her choices for care, telling her that "those pages are not important now." The medical folks can't always make the decisions they think are best, but they do leverage the family to make them. The result was stripping her of her right to make her own healthcare decisions.

Jennie and Janet never fought for a treatment or medication that was not regularly provided to others with her condition(s). In the week before she died, the local hospital never said that the insurance company would not pay for something. They knew they couldn't pull that one anymore because Jennie would call the insurance company and catch the administration in yet another attempted clerical error.

Janet's death happened as it did, in part, because the science of medicine is too good at keeping us alive, we don't take the time to understand its implications and we fail to make truly informed choices about our care at the end. The medical folks are then forced to do the only thing they can, patient manage the family into making what they think are the correct choices. The locals knew that Janet was dying, that she wanted to fight and could well make her own decisions. They also knew that hers was a losing battle, so they worked, with the unknowing assistance of Janet's family, to alter her choices in what they believed to be a medically acceptable way. The process skirts the edge of moral values and ethical standards while violating patient rights (and state laws). Nobody really sees or understands what is happening. The staff and administration played it perfectly. Janet was not the first patient to have their healthcare choices reworked at the last minute.

⌒

The real kicker for me is that even when everyone knew she was not going to live any longer, she was not allowed to die in her own home. Janet's house was fully equipped for her to go home. She had essentially a hospital room in her house. She had every home respiratory aid and Jennie had been trained in all of it. When they took her off the respirator, she was not given oxygen and was able to breathe on her own for another day. There is little doubt that Janet could have come home with oxygen, survived a few more days and died in the warmth of her own home with all of her family around her. Even if she had died on the ride home, at least she would have known that we attempted to honor her choice.

⌒

Whenever I talk about what I do for work I get one of three responses. A good number go directly into sharing stories about their experiences and challenges with their parents currently or in the past. With some folks, the topic rings a bell and they want to know more, when our next class is or to make an appointment. The others that I talk to about healthcare advocacy express regret at not stepping up and engaging in their parents care. They don't always fess up and state that they wish they were currently or that they wished they had helped their parents before they died. Some just get a faraway look in their eyes and lower their voice when offering some justification for not having done so. From that less than scientific analysis, it is clear to me that everyone helps Mom and Dad, wants to or ends up feeling guilty when they don't. You'll be doing Mom, Dad, and yourself a huge favor, just jump in and do the best you can. Help them with their healthcare and deaths. If you do, you will share a loving and rewarding experience that can't be expressed in words. When you don't, regardless of what you think of your relationship with Mom or Dad, you'll miss an opportunity for growth like few others.

⁓

We hope some of what you've read in this book will help you as you care for your parents, but the ideas and strategies you've read do not even scratch the surface. Every person that has taken care of their mother has good ideas for you also, talk about it with them. They have just as many lessons and horror stories as Jennie and I. With our aging population blooming the way it is, you're never standing very far from someone whose parents need them and they're just as unsure of how to help them as you are yours. Talking about being our parents' healthcare advocate really is where the end begins.

You have your own way of doing things. Mom and Dad need your help. You really should do something. The thoughts and processes in this book are proven to work. It doesn't matter whether you focus your effort around our methods, craft your own, or go with a combination, you need to be prepared and consistent. If you won't do both, be consistent. Consistent both with the time you spend talking with your parents, being with them and your efforts in dealing with the medical folks.

*The End*

# Afterword

IF YOU WOULD LIKE to know more or wish to contact Jennie and I, please visit our website www.helpingourparentsbook.com.

Jennie and I also offer Healthcare Advocacy consulting services in all 50 states and are available for speaking engagements as well. I am licensed to provide Healthcare Advocacy centered legal services in Maine, New Hampshire and Massachusetts.

# Disclaimer

As a reader of this book, please know that neither Mike nor Jennie are certified or working professionals in the medical industry. The events, stories, situations and teachings from which you will read and learn come from our combined years of experience caring and advocating as a son & daughter; primary caregivers of other loved ones and friends; and, the wealth of knowledge learned from interfacing with medical professionals in many different states and different medical facilities. It was our goal to pass this information on to you in the greatest hope that it may help prevent or eliminate the repeat of the bad performances for you and your parents and applaud those servicing angels who care for our loved ones unyielded by the ever changing business of the medical industry.

# Works Cited

1    "Thanksgiving." *Blue Bloods,* created by Robin Green and Mitchell
     Burgess, performance by Tom Selleck, season 2, episode 8, CBS
     Television Studios, November 18, 2011.

2    Goldman, Brian Dr. *The Secret Language of Doctors Cracking the Code of
     Hospital Culture.* Illinois: Triumph Books, LLC. 2014. 108-109.

3    Groopman, Jerome M.D. *How Doctors Think.* New York: First Mariner
     Books. 2008. Chapter 5 (101-131).

4    Byock, Ira MD *The Best Care Possible.* New York: Avery. Penquin Group.
     2013. 224-227.

5    Byock, Ira, M.D. *Dying Well Peace and Possibilities at the End of Life.*
     NewYork: Riverhead Books, Berkley Publishing Group, a division of
     Penquin Putnam, Inc. 1997. 247.

6    Volandes, Angelo E. *The Conversation A Revolutionary Plan for End-of-
     Life Care.* New York: Bloomsbury. 2015. 6,27,30.

7    Katz, Jay. *The Silent World of Doctor and Patient.* Baltimore: The John
     Hopkins University Press. 2002. 130

8    Gawande, Atul *Being Mortal Medicine and What Matters in the End.* New
     York: Metropolitan Books Henry Holt and Company, LLC. 2014. 197

9    Katz, Jay. *The Silent World of Doctor and Patient.* Baltimore: The John
     Hopkins University Press. 2002. xxxii

10   45 C.F.R § 164.524(c).

11   New Hampshire Law RSA 137-J: 18.

12   Katz, Jay. *The Silent World of Doctor and Patient*. Baltimore: The John Hopkins University Press. 2002. 88,100,104

13   Aldridge, Melissa D., and Amy S. Kelley. "The Myth Regarding the High Cost of End-of-Life Care." *American Journal of Public Health* 105.12 (2015): 2411–2415. *PMC*. Web. 19 Apr. 2017.

14   Goldman, Brian Dr. *The Secret Language of Doctors Cracking the Code of Hospital Culture*. Illinois: Triumph Books, LLC. 2014. 320.

15   Volandes, Angelo E. *The Conversation A Revolutionary Plan for End-of-Life Care*. New York: Bloomsbury. 2015. 57.

16   https://www.mayoclinic.org/home/ovc-20336882

17   Nuland, Sherwin B., *How We Die Reflections on Life's Final Chapter*. New York: Vintage Books, A Division of Random House, Inc. 1995. 222, 223, 228, 231, 233, 236.

18   https://csupalliativecare.org/palliativecommunity/what-is-palliative-care/

19   https://www.cms.gov/Outreach-and-Education/Medicare-Learning-Network-MLN/MLNProducts/Downloads/AdvanceCarePlanning.pdf

20   http://cpr.heart.org/AHAECC/CPRAndECC/General/UCM_477263_Cardiac-Arrest-Statistics.jsp

21   Yuen, Jacqueline K., M. Carrington Reid, and Michael D. Fetters. "Hospital Do-Not-Resuscitate Orders: Why They Have Failed and How to Fix Them." *Journal of General Internal Medicine* 26.7 (2011): 791–797. *PMC*. Web. 8 Nov. 2017.

22   Goldman, Brian Dr. *The Secret Language of Doctors Cracking the Code of Hospital Culture*. Illinois: Triumph Books, LLC. 2014. 308, 310.

23   http://www.themha.org/policy-advocacy/Issues/End-of-Life-Care/advdirectivesform.aspx

24   Byock, Ira, M.D. *Dying Well Peace and Possibilities at the End of Life*. NewYork: Riverhead Books, Berkley Publishing Group, a division of Penquin Putnam, Inc. 1997. 32.

25   https://www.genworth.com/about-us/industry-expertise/cost-of-care. html.

26   http://www.folife.org/

27   45 CFR 160, 162, and 164

28   Butler, Katy. *Knocking on Heaven's Door The Path to a Better Way of Death.* New York: Scribner A Division of Simon & Schuster, Inc. 2013. 3, 12, 47, 49

29   Groopman, Jerome M.D. *How Doctors Think.* New York: First Mariner Books. 2008. 17.

30   Goldman, Brian Dr. *The Secret Language of Doctors Cracking the Code of Hospital Culture.* Illinois: Triumph Books, LLC. 2014. 82.

31   Miller, Robert H. and Bissell, Daniel M. M.D. *Med School Confidential A Complete Guide to the Medical School Experience: By Students, for Students* New York: Thomas Dunne Books St. Martin's Griffin. 2006. xvii & xviii.

32   Miller, Robert H. and Bissell, Daniel M. M.D. *Med School Confidential A Complete Guide to the Medical School Experience: By Students, for Students* New York: Thomas Dunne Books St. Martin's Griffin. 2006. 177.

33   Groopman, Jerome M.D. *How Doctors Think.* New York: First Mariner Books. 2008. 4-5.

34   https://www.guideline.gov/

35   Goldman, Brian Dr. *The Secret Language of Doctors Cracking the Code of Hospital Culture.* Illinois: Triumph Books, LLC. 2014. 280.

36   http://www.medicalarchives.jhmi.edu/osler/aequessay.htm

37   Volandes, Angelo E. *The Conversation A Revolutionary Plan for End-of-Life Care.* New York: Bloomsbury. 2015. 27.

38   Brown, Theresa *Critical Care A New Nurse Faces Death, Life, and Everything in Between* New York: Harper One HarperCollins Publishers. 2011. 63, 66, 144.

39  http://www.georgecarlin.net/quotes.html

40  http://news.gallup.com/businessjournal/195209/few-millennials-engaged-work.aspx http://news.gallup.com/poll/180404/gallup-daily-employee-engagement.aspx

41  Haudan, Jim CEO, Root Learning *The Art of Engagement*. New York: McGraw Hill .2008.

42  Goldman, Brian Dr. *The Secret Language of Doctors Cracking the Code of Hospital Culture.* Illinois: Triumph Books, LLC. 2014. 78.

43  Groopman, Jerome M.D. *How Doctors Think*. New York: First Mariner Books. 2008. 67.

44  Groopman, Jerome M.D. *How Doctors Think*. New York: First Mariner Books. 2008. 75, 263.

45  https://www.merriam-webster.com/dictionary/confabulate

46  Groopman, Jerome M.D. *How Doctors Think*. New York: First Mariner Books. 2008. 267.

47  Katz, Jay. *The Silent World of Doctor and Patient.* Baltimore: The John Hopkins University Press. 2002. 213.

48  Byock, Ira, M.D. *Dying Well Peace and Possibilities at the End of Life.* NewYork: Riverhead Books, Berkley Publishing Group, a division of Penquin Putnam, Inc. 1997. 43.

49  Nuland, Sherwin B., *How We Die Reflections on Life's Final Chapter.* New York: Vintage Books, A Division of Random House, Inc. 1995. 248.

50  Byock, Ira, M.D. *Dying Well Peace and Possibilities at the End of Life.* NewYork: Riverhead Books, Berkley Publishing Group, a division of Penquin Putnam, Inc. 1997. 25-26, 30-31.